OVERCOMING
HEADACHES

A

NATURAL

APPROACH

Pat Thomas

D1526430

THE CROSSING PRESS
FREEDOM, CALIFORNIA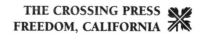

For information on bulk purchases or group discounts for this and other
Crossing Press titles, please contact our Special Sales Manager at
800/777-1048.

Visit our Web site: **www.crossingpress.com**

Library of Congress Cataloging-in-Publication Data

Thomas, Pat, 1959-
    [Headaches]
    Overcoming headaches : a natural approach / Pat Thomas.
       p. cm.
    Includes bibliographical references and index.
    ISBN 1-58091-105-6 (pbk.)
    1.Headache--Popular works. 2. Headache--Alternative treatment.
      I. Title.

RC392.T48 2001
616.8'491--dc21

                      00-050946

0   9   8   7   6   5   4   3   2   1

TABLE OF CONTENTS

CHAPTER 1

What Are Headaches?

Headaches are among the oldest and most common health complaints of the human race. The subtle and not-so-subtle levels of pain can range from the dull throbbing of a tension headache to the nausea, flashing lights, and drilling sensation of a classic migraine. The pain can last minutes, hours—even days; it can debilitate or, according to legend, inspire.

For instance, some people believe that the flashing light in the Bible story of Saul's conversion to Paul may have been a migraine aura. In later years, Paul became a great preacher and writer, transcending the often painful headaches and visual problems which would plague him for the rest of his life.

The weird trip that Alice took in Wonderland gave her a headache. But could Lewis Carroll, the author, who was also a migraine sufferer, ever have imagined that one day other migraine sufferers would suffer what is called an "Alice in Wonderland" syndrome—feeling parts of their body growing or shrinking to odd shapes and sizes and seeing things which are not there?

Headaches are not a modern dilemma. In the Stone Age, pieces of a headache sufferer's skull were cut away with flint instruments in order to relieve the pain. The ancient Egyptians blamed headaches on an invasion by evil spirits and treated them with a mixture of herbs and opium. In 400 B.C. Hippocrates, the father of modern medicine, described the course of a migraine clearly. Around the time of the birth of Christ, physicians bled their patients and then applied a hot iron to the site of the pain. They also made incisions in the person's temple into which they inserted raw garlic. When that failed, they sometimes tried applying electric eels (living and dead) directly to the head. Two centuries later in Alexandria, the physician Aretaeus labeled migraines as hemierania because of their effect on one side of the head. Around the Ninth Century in the British Isles, one headache remedy involved drinking the juice of elderseed, cow's brain, and goat's dung dissolved in vinegar.

The remedy sounds unpleasant, but it couldn't have been much worse than the side effects of some modern "cures." One new headache drug can cause severe chest pain, heart attack, flushing, dizziness, weakness, altered liver function, nausea, and vomiting. Another can cause similar so-called side effects and has in some cases made headaches worse. Even aspirin, taken in large quantities over long periods of time, can cause intestinal bleeding and kidney damage. We are still a long way from providing effective relief from the wide variety of commonly experienced headaches.

Almost anyone can get a headache—there is evidence that nine out of ten adults have suffered a headache at some time in their life. Women, children, and the elderly are more prone to headaches than men are. We don't know why. Normal hormonal fluctuations may possibly be linked to women's chronic headaches, but there is no real evidence to substantiate this. Children's lives are often more stressful than most adults imagine—they also have a much stronger mind/body connection. Headaches in the elderly are not a normal part of aging; in part, it may be due to the quantity of prescription drugs the elderly take as a matter of course.

While we are still a long way from fully understanding the mechanism of headaches, we do know that headaches, including migraines, are not in themselves disorders but instead are symptoms of some other problem. Find the problem and you will find the solution—or the beginning of a solution—to your headache pain.

One of the most effective ways to find the problem is to become a headache detective. No one else can do this for you. No one else lives in your body and knows your pattern of symptoms and pain as well as you do. Even your doctor will not be as precise as you are. You hold the key. By making yourself aware of the circumstances which can trigger your headache by keeping a headache diary (see Chapter 3), you are on the road to relieving your headache pain and the disruptive effect it has on your life.

Many people worry that headache pain needs to be treated immediately. This may discourage them from taking the time to hunt for the cause of the pain. One of the big misconceptions about headaches is that the longer you have had them, the more likely it is that there is something seriously wrong with you. Actually, the opposite is true. Very severe headaches that come on suddenly—those caused by meningitis, stroke, or a sub-arachnoid hemorrhage—are the most dangerous. These are thankfully rare. Long-term, chronic headaches may be painful and disruptive, but they are generally not life-threatening.

Pain is your body's way of telling you something is wrong.

Usually it starts in the nervous system as a result of irritation or inflammation. A complex system of nerve fibers conveys the message of pain to the brain, and the brain responds immediately by sending out an instruction to avoid the source of the pain. For instance, if you burn your finger, your brain tells you to take your hand away from the fire; if you stepped on a stone, your brain would say it's time to put your shoes on.

Pain is essentially a messenger. When we blast the pain with pain-killing drugs, we are in effect shooting the messenger instead of listening to the message. This prevents us from taking appropriate, long-term protective action. While there is a legitimate place in the treatment of headaches for many conventional drugs, we often pay a high price when we take such drugs routinely. We often end up trading one set of distressing symptoms for another. If the occasional headache responds to simple pain-relieving drugs such as aspirin, great. But it is important to remember that aspirin, like most drugs, can only suppress symptoms. These drugs do not address the cause of chronic pain.

In simple terms you could say that the majority of headaches are caused by some form of stress. Stress certainly may have an emotional origin—it's the first thing most of us think of when we hear the word. But stress can have a physical foundation as well. For example, your body can be under stress from an oncoming viral infection, a food allergy, a chemical sensitivity, or a spinal misalignment.

Tension headaches are the most common type—most people suffer from these at some point in their lives. Figures show that more than fifty percent of headache sufferers never report their symptoms to a doctor or seek any outside help. We tend to shrug off a tension headache as unimportant. It's probably best not to complain, just take two aspirin and forget about it. Even if your headache is not triggered by stress, the chronic pain which a headache can bring can create stress in your life and the problem can become self-perpetuating.

Too often in our culture we try to ignore stress and numb the pain, whatever its source, rather than becoming familiar with it. And yet, it is familiarity which eventually allows us to begin to track down the real cause of headache pain.

The truth is, you are probably your own best general practitioner when it comes to treating your headache, since only you will know what the pain feels like, when it generally comes on, and what makes it worse or better. Although many headache sufferers feel as if they have no options and no hope of relief, there is a wide range of alternative therapies and self-help options available. Pursuing these options provides genuine relief from headache pain, and also will give you a sense that you have achieved something for yourself. This latter point is important, since so many headache sufferers feel at the mercy of both their bodies and the medications aimed at controlling their symptoms.

In order to solve the riddle of your headache, you first need to educate yourself about all the potential causes and your options for treatment. Then you should consider seeking out those practitioners who believe in treating the body as a whole.

Because headaches are so common, and because conventional medicine has such a poor track record in relieving them, there has been plenty of research into alternative therapies such as herbs, chiropractic, aromatherapy, or homeopathy. Since many doctors feel frustrated by their inability to help chronic headache sufferers, they may even be pleased to see their patients taking the initiative and investigating other options!

Although you have all the clues to your headache pain inside you, making sense of what you already know can be difficult. This is where an alternative practitioner may prove a helpful companion. Most alternative therapists are skilled in the art of history taking—an art which many GPs have lost or don't have time to practice. This is exactly what will enable both you and your practitioner to track down the cause of your headache. The two of you can begin to piece together these seemingly unrelated bits of information, until eventually the picture of what triggers your headache becomes clear.

Headaches can occur for many different reasons and need to be treated according to their cause. Headache pain can be caused by factors unrelated to the head itself. It can be what is known as referred pain, caused by digestive disorders or pelvic irritation and transferred to corresponding areas in the head, where it is experienced as head pain. A good practitioner will know this and search for the real cause of your headache, instead of just handing you a prescription for something to (temporarily) take away the pain.

Alternative medicine treats you as a whole person. This is important, since a headache is more than a pain in the head. It is not a disease, but a symptom of something else. Finding that something else is what you and your alternative practitioner can do as a team.

CHAPTER 2

What Type of Headache?

Depending on what research you read, there can be anything from three to three hundred different types of headache. Why so many? Because headaches are a particularly complex health problem. By putting labels to the many variations of headache pain, researchers have been better able to understand the many types of triggers. The problem is that the symptoms of one type of headache overlap with the symptoms of another. And while most people tend to suffer from one type of headache or another, some people suffer from several different types. An example would be a person who has arthritis of the neck, muscular tension, and migraine.

Labeling headache types also creates problems because it encourages a particularly unhelpful kind of diagnostic pigeonholing. So, today, instead of treating people as individuals and recognizing that while broad patterns exist, each individual responds slightly differently to headache triggers (and some don't respond at all), we treat them as labels, or as headache types.

There is even a good argument that all headaches are related, inasmuch as they all stem from either metabolic, structural, and/or emotional stress. Nevertheless, the experience of pain is entirely individual, and other factors, such as whether you are able to rest, your work or home environment, and even the weather can profoundly affect the course of a headache once it has started.

What follows are brief descriptions of the most common types of headaches. However, as you read, try not to get too bogged down by the labels; look instead at the bigger picture to see if any of the symptoms resonate with your personal situation. Each section contains a summary of common triggers for each type of headache, which may give you new possibilities to explore as you begin to search for the causes and cures for your own pain.

TENSION HEADACHES

This is probably the most common type of headache, accounting for four out of five visits to a physician. Chances are, if your headache isn't an obvious migraine or a cluster headache, your doctor is likely to tell you that you are suffering from a tension headache. Today, it has become something of a meaningless, catch-all diagnosis which tells you little, if anything, about the origin of your pain. What is more, the name tension headache can be misleading, since to many people it suggests an emotional/psychological root to the problem.

Some doctors use the term muscle contraction headache instead, though this is not much more helpful. A better description would be a stress-induced headache; in this case, anything which puts the body and/or mind under stress can be the cause. This can include repressed emotions, poor food, constipation, insomnia, and hormonal changes. Stress factors may also include chemical pollution at home or at work.

Some people experience this type of headache on a daily basis. There are contractions of the muscles in the scalp, and the pain starts at the base of the neck and spreads over the top of the head and onto the forehead. Often it feels like a heavy weight is pressing down on your head, or a tight band is constricting it. Sometimes not all of the scalp muscles are involved, so the pain can be localized to just one area just above the eyes.

Muscle contraction is the result, not the cause, of the headache. That is, anything that strains the muscles in the neck or scalp can trigger this type of headache. Fatigue, unhealthy working conditions, poor posture, or staying in the same position for long periods of time are all contributing factors. Tension headaches are common after long car or plane rides. They are frequently found in computer programmers, secretaries—anyone who has to work in poorly designed chairs. As this type of headache becomes more and more common, whole industries of chair manufacturers have sprung up claiming to have scientifically designed, ergonomic seating for home and office. Nevertheless, the problem persists.

Although tension headaches can be caused by a baffling variety of different things, the good news is that once you find the trigger or triggers, it is relatively easy to stop the pain.

MIGRAINE

A migraine is not a headache, but a whole disease process. Clinically it is defined as a specific disease of the nervous system, which produces a one-sided headache, vomiting, and occasionally flashing lights in front of the eye. Roughly one in ten people suffer from this type of disorder, which can disrupt much of their life at home and at work. Women are three times more likely to suffer from migraines than men. Children are also susceptible to migraines, though often they do not suffer them in the same way as adults. In a child, sometimes the migraine is felt in the head and at other times in the stomach (see Chapter 13).

Although migraines can be defined by a broad range of symptoms, they also appear to be very individualized, with symptom patterns varying from person to person. Migraines can be debilitating and come on quickly, bringing a range of unpleasant symptoms and a pain which is often described as like having someone drill a hole through your head.

It is a misconception that migraines are an intellectual's disorder—they strike people from every kind of background. Nor are they a neurotic condition. The pain of a migraine comes from the dilation, or widening, of the blood vessels in the lower part of the brain. This is what brings about the characteristic throbbing sensation. Dilation is often—though not always—preceded by a contraction, or narrowing, of the same blood vessels. It is this which is thought to produce the visual problems which sometimes occur before the actual headache. The alternate widening and narrowing of the blood vessels puts pressure on the nerve endings and causes irritation, which in turn causes the headache.

While it sounds relatively straightforward on paper, these changes occur in response to a variety of complex chemical changes within the body. For instance, it is now believed that migraine sufferers—and to a lesser extent those who suffer from tension and cluster headaches—may have an imbalance in an important brain chemical called serotonin. Serotonin influences our sense of well-being, but an excess of it can also cause the blood vessels to contract. An imbalance of such chemicals within the brain can be triggered by a variety of external factors. Stress is one, but equally, hormonal fluctuations, changes in weather and altitude, bright lights, loud noises, disturbed sleep patterns, and pollution all play their part. But more and more we are beginning to see that diet, or more specifically food intolerance and allergy, plays a major part in the development of migraine.

Although we tend to think of migraines as a single entity, there are variations of the type of headache they bring. The most widely experienced form is the one-sided, pulsating headache, lasting between one and three days. This is usually accompanied by vomiting and nausea and a sensitivity to light and noise. Between attacks, the sufferers will usually experience complete freedom from pain and other symptoms. This is the common migraine.

The classical form of migraine displays all the same symptoms as the common migraine, but also has what is called an aura beforehand, which can last up to an hour. An aura is an inexplicable feeling or sensation which warns the sufferer that he or she is about to have another attack. Often an aura is accompanied by visual disturbances, which can produce a halo effect around objects.

Some migraines follow predictable phases. There is the prodrome phase, where there may be food cravings, yawning, irritability, or euphoria; the aura, with flashing lights in front of the eyes, blind spots in the field of vision, numbness or difficulty speaking properly; the headache phase, during which the pain strikes, along with other symptoms such as nausea, vomiting, and sensitivity to light and sound; the resolution phase, during which the symptoms begin to ebb and the sufferer is able to sleep it off; and the recovery phase, which is characterized by exhaustion and a feeling of being totally washed out. This is a complete migraine, though not all migraine sufferers experience every part of the cycle. Migraines don't always produce severe pain, are not always disabling, and do not have to occur frequently. Some people have weekly attacks and others may suffer only one or two a year. These details are unimportant in migraine diagnosis. It is the symptoms, not their severity or frequency, which define a migraine.

CLUSTER HEADACHES

A close relative of the migraine, this is a one-sided headache that produces a stabbing pain behind one eye with weeping and redness of that eye. There may also be facial flushing, drooping of the eyelids, sweating, and nasal congestion. Attacks last between fifteen minutes to three hours. They tend to come in clusters (thus the name) over a period of weeks. Typically, there will be pain-free periods in between attacks, but these rarely last longer than three hours in any cycle. Cluster headaches affect four times as many men as women.

It is believed that cluster headaches are linked in some way with seasonal changes. Most attacks, for instance, occur in spring and autumn, when daylight hours are undergoing transition. But cluster headaches also have a biochemical basis. Anything which throws the normal body chemistry out of balance is a likely contributor. This can include alcohol, heavy smoking, cold wind or hot air blowing across the face, dream-filled sleep, and foods containing amines, which can dilate the blood vessels (see Chapter 5).

Sensitivities and allergies vary from individual to individual, and almost anything can cause an allergic reaction in someone, somewhere. Sensitivity headaches usually occur between four to twelve hours after contact with the offending substance. They manifest as a dull, aching, generalized pain.

This type of headache is a variation of a tension headache and can be caused by single or multiple allergens.

While a great deal of attention has been paid in the media recently to food-related allergens, less attention has been paid to environmental allergens. These can include passive smoke, car pollution, household cleaning products, perfumes, and the gases released from carpets, wallpaper, and plastic items in the home and office. As our homes and offices become more and more safeguarded against the weather, we seal in these toxins, which can, in turn, cause chronic illness with headache symptoms.

Sensitivity/allergy headaches are among the easiest to cure. Symptoms usually begin to disappear once you have identified the allergen and removed it from your diet or environment. Many people are surprised at how much better they feel generally once this is done. They have an immediate surge of energy and a greater interest in life. In some individuals, however, healing can be slow if there has been a long-term toxic build-up in the body.

SINUS HEADACHES

If you suffer from frequent colds or live in a polluted area, you are likely to experience sinus congestion and the aching pain in the front of your face. This sinus headache is closely related to the sensitivity/allergy headache and often has the same triggers. The sinuses are hollow, air-filled spaces in the cheekbones and the bones of the forehead. These cavities are connected to the nose via narrow channels, and their main function is to produce mucus for the nasal passages. This fluid protects the lungs by trapping any foreign particles that are breathed in. If the sinuses are irritated, either from pollutants or a cold, they secrete more mucus. This excess mucus should flow down the narrow channels to the nose, but often these channels are blocked and inflamed for the same reason that the sinuses are irritated. Stagnation of the mucus leads to infection and to increased pressure in the sinus cavities. As these are surrounded by bone, they are unable to expand to ease the pressure and become quite tender and painful. This is why sufferers often feel an intense throbbing behind or above the eyes.

The most common triggers for sinus headaches are pollen, dust, cigarette smoke, and pollution (indoor and outdoor). But since the sinuses can also become inflamed as a result of an allergic reaction, you should also consider foods and household chemicals as potential triggers.

DENTAL HEADACHES

With this type of headache the cause is in the mouth. An abnormal bite, grinding your teeth as you sleep (often as a result of stress and worry), and dental infection can lead to headaches. The pain is usually felt in the jaw and around the mouth, but can spread to the temples. If your jaw makes a popping, clicking, or cracking sound when eating and/or if pain and tenderness come on after eating or yawning, this is a sign of jaw misalignment. This type of headache is generally less severe than other types. It can be treated by dentistry and occasionally manual therapies such as chiropractic and osteopathy.

EYESTRAIN HEADACHES

The eyes are mostly muscle and they can become fatigued from overuse just like any other muscle of the body. Persistent eyestrain can be caused by working in conditions of poor lighting, or perhaps by the need for corrective lenses. Sometimes they are the result of wearing your glasses when you don't really need to, thus forcing your eyes to remain at a fixed focus for long periods of time.

There usually is only one trigger—overusing your eyes in some way. Eyestrain headache can be brought on by long periods of focused visual work such as working at a computer, doing detailed art work, reading books for too long or in poor light, or working in a room with overhead fluorescent lighting. The one exception to these triggers is that a headache around the eyes can also be a case of referred pain—where the pain travels from one site to another before it is felt—caused by digestive disturbances and misalignment of the spine or joints.

TRAUMA HEADACHE

It may seem obvious that if you bang your head it will hurt. However, a trauma headache can also be the result of referred pain, and damage to the spine or other areas of the body can end up giving you a headache.

With a trauma headache sometimes there is a delayed reaction, so you may not feel the pain resulting from trauma immediately. But once it strikes it can become a regular feature in your life for years afterward. In addition, the pain you feel may bear little relation to the injury you received. Even small blows to the head can cause severe, recurrent headaches for a long time afterward.

Once it does surface, headache pain from trauma can occur daily and be resistant to treatment. It may be accompanied by dizziness or nausea, moodiness, insomnia, fatigue, and shortened attention span. Spinal manipulation such as osteopathy or chiropractic are often the most helpful therapies in these cases.

EXERTION HEADACHE

As the name suggests, this type of headache usually follows exertion such as coughing, sneezing, or a strained bowel movement. One classic example of an exertion headache is the headache which comes on after sex. It may sound like a joke, but the exertion of lovemaking, combined with the muscular contraction of the head and neck muscles during sexual excitement or orgasm, can end up causing a particularly severe head pain.

Exertion headaches are vascular in nature—a swelling of the arteries and veins in turn makes the blood vessels in the head swell. They are fairly easy to treat with dietary changes, relaxation techniques, and manual manipulation.

REBOUND HEADACHE

Among the elderly, headaches are common—but how often do we stop to consider that these headaches may be a side effect of medication use, not a symptom of something inherently wrong? When a headache is the result of medication (or the overuse of any substance), it is called a rebound headache. Medications which commonly cause headaches include those used to treat heart conditions and diabetes.

Overuse of paracetamol can also cause chronic headaches. Ironically, ergotamine, a drug commonly used for migraine, can also cause a rebound effect. Ergotamine is a vasoconstrictor; in other words, it narrows the blood vessels. Excessive use of this drug can create circulatory problems and changes in the heart rate or blood pressure, which can result in more frequent and more severe headaches. Moreover, users can become quite dependent on the drug and experience withdrawal symptoms when first coming off it. On withdrawal from any migraine medicine containing ergotamine, you may experience quite severe headaches, though these will gradually decrease as the drug clears out of your system.

You can also get rebound headaches as you reduce the toxic load on your body. For instance, rebound headaches are a common symptom in people who decide to give up caffeine. Foods which contain caffeine constrict blood vessels. The eventual "rebound" dilation can give you a headache. Rebound headaches are best treated by gradually removing the rebound-causing substance and detoxifying the body. Once your body adjusts, the rebound headache usually goes away.

A final cause of rebound headache is emotional/mental stress. This type of headache is often difficult to diagnose, because it happens after the level of stress has been reduced. This is very common, for instance, in busy executives who seem to cope quite well with their hectic schedules all week and then, once the pressure is off, are incapacitated by headaches on the weekend.

ORGANIC HEADACHES

Although this is potentially the most serious type of headache, it is also the most rare, which is why I put it last in the list. The organic headache is the one everybody fears, but which very few people actually have. It comes from brain tumors and infections such as meningitis. This type of headache constitutes only one or two percent of all headaches. This is a serious headache and should be ruled out to your satisfaction before you begin any treatment for headache pain. In general, the pain of an organic headache comes on suddenly, will occur daily, and can be made worse through exertion or coughing.

Any new type of head pain which is not relieved by sleeping or wakes you up at night and may be accompanied by bleeding from the nose, mouth, or ear should be taken very seriously and investigated by your doctor.

CHAPTER 3

Tracking Down the Cause

Our major body systems are so finely balanced it does not take much to change bearable stress into unbearable stress. Too much stress inevitably causes our bodies to cease functioning properly, and when this happens, the body sends out warning signals in the form of headaches and other symptoms.

In order to understand what stress does to your body, you will need a basic understanding of how your body functions and the roles each of the major body systems—the digestive, endocrine (hormonal), and nervous systems—plays in keeping you healthy.

Our major body systems protect us from stress and from illness. When one system is working poorly due to outside influences or to poor maintenance, illness with headache symptoms can follow.

THE DIGESTIVE SYSTEM

What you eat and how you eat play a big part in your overall health. In a healthy person, digestion starts as soon as food enters your mouth. The saliva which you produce while chewing begins to break down your food, so that it will be easier to digest once it reaches the stomach. The stomach's digestive juices liquefy and process the food further so that it can move into the intestines, where the essential nutrient and non-nutrient components are extracted.

Several things can interfere with the process of digestion. Eating too much, eating too quickly, and eating the wrong foods may cause the system to break down. These are the foods you may be sensitive or allergic to, those which are highly processed, those which include preservatives and additives, and those which are high in sugar and fat.

These foods may damage the intestinal wall, making it unable to extract the nutrients from your food. High and regular consumption of these foods can lead to a condition called the leaky gut syndrome, where the walls of the intestines which function as a barrier and gatekeeper become damaged and begin to let toxins and other irritants into the bloodstream. Once this happens, your immune system becomes overstimulated and acts as if it were under attack by these foreign particles. One of the body's reactions to this irritation is a chronic headache. Even if your gut is more or less intact, poor digestion can mean that you are not absorbing many of the essential nutrients you need to maintain good health.

THE ENDOCRINE SYSTEM

We tend to think of hormones in a very limited way, our perception being that they only govern our sexual characteristics. However, the word hormone comes from a Greek word meaning "to set into action." Hormones are very powerful chemical messengers which guide and regulate most of the body's chemistry, normalizing and integrating all our bodily functions. They provide a kind of blueprint which determines how tall we are, the distribution of hair and body fat, how our voices sound, our emotional patterns, and the type and location of pain.

When toxic substances enter the bloodstream and begin to irritate the major organs and tissues of the body, the endocrine system is also affected. It goes into overdrive so that it can assist in detoxifying the body before it becomes too weak to defend itself.

As a side note, hormonal changes associated with the menstrual cycle are a contributing factor in some women's headaches. Many women accept without question the diagnosis of "hormonal imbalance" as if it was merely part of their cycle. It is not. If a woman can link her headache with her monthly cycle, that's only the first step in detective work. The next step is to consider all the reasons why her hormonal system may be out of balance. The cause is likely to be diet, environment, and lifestyle rather than hormones.

THE NERVOUS SYSTEM

The nervous system is comprised of the brain, spinal chord, and nerve fibers, plus the chemical messengers which help the various areas of the body communicate with each other. These chemical messengers are called neurotransmitters; the two most important ones with regard to headache pain are serotonin and endorphins.

Serotonin affects our sense of well-being and also regulates the diameter of blood vessels, smooth digestive muscle operation, moods, and reactions to stress. Endorphins lessen our perception of pain and regulate transmission of messages between the nerves. Other key neurotransmitters which are involved in our perception of pain include dopamine, norepinephrine, and acetylcholine. When the production and function of these messengers is blocked due to some toxic build-up or stress, headache can result.

STRESS REVISITED

Broadly speaking, there are three sources of stress—digestive, mental/emotional, and environmental—which can stop your body from working optimally and eventually cause illness. Ways to deal with each kind of stress are discussed at greater length in the chapters which follow, but an overview may be helpful as you embark on the task of looking for the cause of your headache.

DIGESTIVE STRESS

Digestive stress is a very common source of headaches. It can be caused by something as simple as eating a meal too quickly, or eating too much, so that the body cannot digest it properly. Or it can be caused by eating something you are allergic to. Many of us consume much more food than we need. If we do so, we never give our digestive systems a chance to rest and repair. Instead, they are overworked, having to process an over-abundance of food.

According to the Chinese, the head is a compact representation of the digestive system, and head pain always points to a corresponding point in the digestive system. In traditional Chinese medicine the forehead, for instance, is related to the intestines; the side of the head to the liver, gallbladder, and circulation; and the back of the head to the liver and kidneys. Because of the way in which the head is structured, overconsumption of "expansive" foods such as sugar, alcohol, caffeine, and fruit juice is believed to result in pain to the forehead or eyes. A dull, constant pain in the back or side of the head is believed to be the result of "contractive" foods such as meat, eggs, and salt (see Chapter 5).

The typical Western diet is big on quantity and small on quality. We consume far too many processed foods, too much protein, and too few whole grains and fresh fruits and vegetables than our bodies require to stay healthy. Fast foods, however convenient, are the fast track to a variety of health problems. The additives used to give these foods a long shelf-life can cause a toxic build-up in your body, and the lack of essential nutrients can cause vitamin and mineral deficiencies. Denied the proper fuel, your body will eventually start to complain.

Some people believe that in order to compensate for rushed meals and poor-quality food, all you need to do is take a multi-vitamin and mineral supplement. For some this may literally be their only source of essential nutrients. But if your body systems are not working well, it is unlikely that you will be able to absorb and utilize even these prepackaged nutrients. Also, many of the nutritional supplements on the market vary in the quality and quantity of their ingredients, making it hard to guarantee that you are genuinely getting all the nutrients you need. The only real solution is to alter your diet to give your body what it needs to thrive and function optimally.

MENTAL/EMOTIONAL STRESS

Mental/emotional stress has an equally profound effect on your body. Emotions, even the ones we label as negative, are not toxic, but our responses to these emotions can be. Anxiety, depression, repressed anger, and a poor self-image can all leave us fearful and vulnerable. When we feel this way, the body tries to bolster us up, often with a tensing of the muscles.

Muscle tension isn't a meaningless reaction to the stuff that stresses us out. It may serve a genuine purpose in our lives. For example, tense muscles can make you feel stronger or more powerful; they may act like a suit of armor to protect you from harm; they may be the only thing (you think) which is holding you together when you feel like falling apart. Actually, it's hard to stop tensing our muscles precisely because it serves a purpose in our lives. Often we can't let go until we feel safe again, or until we find a better substitute for this painful body armor.

Other physical responses to stress include adrenaline boosts and high blood pressure, which strain the body. The first thing to be affected can be your immune system. Research has indicated that all of our so-called negative emotional states have been linked to a depressed immune system. Chronic headaches may be a message from the rest of your body telling you that you are run-down. A depressed immune system can lead to many more serious diseases, so if you are getting a signal from your body that you need help, take the hint.

ENVIRONMENTAL STRESS

Finally, there is environmental stress, the scope of which scientists and doctors are only just beginning to comprehend. Indoors and out we are subjected to a wide range of chemical irritants and toxins which can adversely affect our health. One of the most common side effects of chemical sensitivity is headache.

Few of us have the choice of living in an unpolluted environment. City dwellers are often obliged to travel, live, and work in places where pollution from cars and factories is a fact of life. Even when we cannot see them, pollutants are all around us in the form of automobile exhaust, pesticides, formaldehydes, radioactive fallout, molds, dust, cigarette smoke, pollens, perfumes, air fresheners, cleaning fluids, and hydrocarbons, to name but a few. People who suffer from chronic headaches tend to be sensitive to all these things.

Don't forget the environment inside your body. Regular use of some medications can pollute your body and end up causing headaches. Most commonly implicated in headache pain are the drugs used to treat high blood pressure, other heart problems, arthritis, and hearing problems. Also included are analgesics, decongestants and other cold medications, oral contraceptives, hormone replacement drugs, antibiotics, antidepressants, and appetite suppressants. If you are taking any of these, speak to your doctor about lowering your dosage or switching to a different medication.

THE WEATHER LINK

Another influential environmental factor is the weather. Migraine sufferers, in particular, report that their symptoms worsen according to what's happening in the weather. While some conservative doctors might think of this as far-fetched, there are writings dating as far back as the eighteenth century describing the relationship between weather and migraine. It was not until 1981 that two researchers, Alan Nusall and David Phillips, began to study the effects of weather on migraine. They discovered that wet, windy, cold weather made the migraine worse, while clear, sunny, dry weather made the migraine more bearable.

A great deal of research has been compiled since then, particularly regarding the role of serotonin in migraine. Nusall speculated that weather's impact on migraine was somehow connected with the body's chemical pain messengers, such as serotonin, prostaglandins, and various other hormonal agents.

In one study of a particularly bitter chinook wind in Canada, women were found to be more sensitive to the changes in weather than men. In another study, when the headache diaries of thirteen patients were analyzed, chinook winds increased the probability of headache onset, particularly in those patients over fifty years old. In another study, forty-three percent of those people who were polled cited weather changes as the trigger for their migraine (second only to stress at sixty-two percent). Strangely, this is an aspect of health often overlooked by doctors, except in Germany, where some physicians are known to make use of daily bulletins from the National Weather Service to advise patients.

I've included the information in this chapter in order to help you become more aware of potential triggers and how they work. Most of the time we aren't aware of the kinds of stress we labor under. We eat food automatically, we shut out the unpleasant aspects of our environment, we ignore our unpleasant emotional impulses. This is why chronic headache sufferers may have to learn to become headache detectives.

A HEADACHE DIARY

When you begin to search for solutions, one of the most helpful things you can do is begin a headache diary. Over the period of a month or so, make careful records of your headaches. Your diary doesn't have to be elaborate, or expensive—a simple, cheap notebook will do—but it does need to be detailed. Consider this diary a consciousness-raising exercise, since you will need to record not only when the headache struck, but everything that happened before and after it stopped. Typically, this would include things like food you ate, the feelings you had, the smells, lights, and sounds you were exposed to, whether you slept the night before, and where you are in your menstrual cycle. Not only will keeping a diary help you, but should you choose to seek the help of a doctor or alternative health practitioner, it will help him or her help you.

Below is a list of things you should include in your headache diary. The first six items will help you establish if there is a regular pattern to your headaches. The remaining items will help you describe your headache pain and are useful for designing a treatment program which suits your individual needs.

The Date and Day of the Week

- Do your headaches occur mainly during the week or on the weekend?
- Does going back to work on Monday precipitate a headache?
- Do your headaches fall on certain days of the week? If so, what are you doing on those days?

The Time of Day

- Did you wake up with a headache? If you did, was it earlier or later than usual?
- Does your headache correspond to a certain time of day, such as before or after eating?
- Did it occur in the morning, afternoon, or evening?

Where Are You in Your Menstrual Cycle?

- Did your headache occur during, before, or after your period?

Where Were You When Your Headache Came On?

- What was your physical environment like? Was it stuffy, smoky, or noisy?
- What was the emotional atmosphere like? Was there any arguing? Was it tense or intimidating?
- Does your headache always begin in the same type of atmosphere?
- Be attentive also to things like smells. Have you been around any new carpeting, furniture, or clothing—all of which are treated with chemicals? Have you been somewhere dusty, moldy, or musty?

What Foods, Beverages, or Medications Had You Taken?

- List everything you ate or drank over the twelve-hour period prior to your headache. If you have a history of headaches, keep a food diary of everything you eat or drink in that period of time. You may find this difficult at first. Eating may be so automatic that remembering can be difficult. With practice, it will get easier.
- If you are taking any medicines, make a note of when and how much you take.

What Were You Doing?

- Your activities on the day your headache occurred may reveal useful information.
- Was the day unusually stressful or upsetting?
- Did you engage in any physically stressful activities?

- Were you doing something which required deep concentration for a long period of time?

How Would You Describe Your Headache?
- Describe the pattern of your headache.
- Describe the type of pain.
- Where is the pain?
- Is it always in the same place? On one or both sides of the head, in the back, front, top of the head, or all over?
- Are other areas painful or sore, such as the neck, upper back, eyes, ears, sinus, jaws?
- Were there any warning signs? For example, did you see lights, colored dots, was there a blind spot, any numbness?
- Have you noticed any problems with your eyes, or been in a situation where your eyes were under strain? Were you using a computer or doing close work all day?
- How painful is your headache? Is it mild, moderate, or severe? Or if you prefer, use a scale of 0 to 10, with 0 being no pain and 10 the worst pain that you have ever had.
- Is the pain constant or throbbing, dull or sharp, generalized, or in a tight band around the head?
- Do you sense the pain as a pressure or radiating to other parts of the body?
- Did your head feel heavy?
- Did it feel as if someone was drilling a hole in it?
- Were there any other symptoms?
- Do any symptoms such as dizziness or light-headedness accompany your headache?
- Do you have nausea, vomiting, diarrhea, nasal stuffiness, or watery eyes?
- Are you sensitive to light? To noise? To touch?

Can You Describe Your Mood?

- At the time the headache began, or during the twenty-four to seventy-two hours preceding it, did you become upset, angry, anxious, worried, bored, or sad? Or were you happy? Remember that some headaches occur after the triggering emotion has passed.

How Long Did Your Headache Last?

- Make a note of how long your headache lasted.
- Was there constant pain throughout that time or did it build up gradually to a peak and then gradually subside?

What Is Your General State of Health at the Moment?

- Headaches don't occur in a vacuum. Place your headache in the context of the total picture of your health.
- Do you suffer from hypertension?
- Are you run-down?

What Made It Better?

- Have you already found a way of getting relief?
- Does an ice pack on the back of the neck or shoulder help?
- Does heat?
- Did you lie down, take a bath or shower?
- Did you engage in some recreational activity?
- Did you take any medication that you found effective?

Your diary should also include anything which might be helpful. For instance, is there any other factor in your headache that was not covered previously? Have you already noticed a pattern which you need to write down?

Once you've come to grips with the information in your

diary, you can start making connections between a potential trigger or triggers and your head pain. You may wish to take your diary and your conclusions to your doctor or alternative practitioner so that he or she can suggest appropriate treatment. Or you may wish to begin a regime of treatments you yourself devise. Even if you have never considered the latter option, with good information about your headache at your fingertips, you are now in a position to choose safely and with confidence from a variety of effective alternatives which are widely available.

CHAPTER 4

Relief from Stress

Stress can produce many different types of diseases. No one is sure why some people react to stress with stomachaches, others with asthma attacks, and others with headaches. Each of our bodies has its own weak spot. It may be that people who get headaches are simply more prone to disorders of this type.

Although stress gets a bad press, not all stress is bad. Our ability to cope with stress is part of what has made humans so successful as a species. The problem is we cope with stress so well that we often fail to notice the build-up of tension in our lives and end up taking on more than we can handle. That's the point where stress turns into strain and begins to be evident in debilitating physical symptoms.

Most people have heard of the fight-or-flight response. When a human is under stress the body produces greater quantities of the hormone adrenaline which helps us by sharpening our wit, and giving us strength and speed. If we were still cave dwellers, we would either fight the threatening animal or marauding neighboring tribe, or run away. But modern society is more complex. Often we are subjected to the sort of stress that we can't defend ourselves from or run away from. For instance, if you disagree with your boss, or if you are confronted with a difficult customer, what can you do?

Sometimes we can't do anything about certain types of stress, such as the rising levels of noise pollution. While society is more complex, our bodies are still pretty much the same as they were hundreds of thousands of years ago. As far as body chemistry is concerned, stress is stress. It makes no difference whether the cause is a wild animal or an outrageous heating bill—the response will be the same.

This automatic chemical response to stress creates problems because unused adrenaline can build up in your system. This causes muscle tension and high blood pressure—both of which are implicated directly and indirectly in a number of disabling conditions, including headaches. In addition to making muscle tension more likely, excess adrenaline can interfere with regular sleep patterns. Unresolved stress can also result in emotional turmoil, which can cause anxiety and depression.

So much of the time we are not even aware of stress. As adults we have learned to shut it out, and we may not even be aware of the way in which our bodies respond to stress, usually by tensing our muscles. Often, we are so used to carrying on regardless that we never stop to notice that our shoulders are hiked up around our ears or that our necks seem to have lost all mobility. Adults in particular adapt very quickly to these tense postures and carry them around like a suit of armor, defending us against the daily onslaught.

It is not possible or even desirable to avoid all stress. However, we can learn to respond to it in ways that are more appropriate. As a first step, you should become more aware of how stress affects you physically and emotionally. With this knowledge, you can begin to take some control over how you manage stress. For instance, you can put a limit on how much stress you can take at home and at work before you take a break—even if it is only five minutes—to breathe, stretch, or meditate.

Anything that puts you under pressure can cause stress and eventually headache. It can come from concentrating on something for too long, or from being bored or under-challenged. It can be emotional, and in this respect is often linked to times we are in transition: moving our homes, getting married, giving birth, having someone we love die.

Recent studies have shown that even the noise from office equipment such as computers can cause stress. The best way to remove the headache is to remove the stress. If the stress is too great or too much a part of our lives, then removing the stress can be a tall order. However, there are several things we can do to take better care of ourselves and to temporarily relieve headaches caused by stressful conditions.

Just as being under pressure can cause a surge of stress-related hormones, relaxation can cause a surge of sedative hormones. This has been demonstrated in studies: blood levels of these hormones and also of brain-wave activity have been measured before and after relaxation and meditation. There is no doubt that you can produce powerful chemical changes in your body simply by taking a five- or ten-minute break. Learning to relax your mind is remarkably easy. You don't need to spend large amounts of money, there is no special clothing you need to wear, and you don't need to affiliate yourself with any organization. You don't need to attend a class, you don't even need to travel. You simply need to learn to cut yourself off from stressful stimuli for as long as it takes to calm things down again. What follows are some quick stress-busting techniques which can easily be incorporated into even the busiest schedules.

DON'T FORGET TO BREATHE

How many times have you been told to take a deep breath and count to ten? The emphasis in our culture is always on getting the air in, even though this is not the most effective way of relieving stress and balancing the emotions. Many practices such as yoga emphasize breathing out—and with good reason. It is the exhalation that takes toxins out of the body and allows all the muscles to release fully and relax. If you are tense, a series of full exhalations will provide quick, effective, and total relaxation.

Surprisingly, many people find it almost impossible to empty their lungs completely when they first try to do so. Panic overtakes them and they gasp for breath and tense their muscles even harder. You may find that it takes practice to learn how to breathe properly, but it's worth persevering. Making a hissing sound as you breathe out may help, As you become better at breathing out fully and in a relaxed way, you can combine breathing practice with guided imagery, perhaps imagining that with each exhalation you are blowing the tension and pain far, far away. Tension headaches respond particularly well to this approach.

PUT IT IN WRITING

Since there is a simple and effective way of putting worries in perspective, invest in a notebook and pen and write them down. Just filing anxieties somewhere other than your mind is often enough to reduce anxiety. Some people make simple lists of all the things which are worrying them. Others find that journal writing, making time each day to write about what they have done, how they are feeling, or what kinds of dreams they are having, is a very good way to stay balanced.

Journal writing in particular provides you with the powerful medicine of hindsight. Over a period of time, as you write about your worries, and also as you write about how you have solved these problems, you often begin to get a sense of perspective about the things you experience on a day-to-day basis. Some of them may even begin to look a bit insignificant after a while. When this happens, it is just a short step to not responding to them in a way which makes you feel ill.

ROCK THE STRESS AWAY

Remember how nice it was to be rocked on your mother's or grandmother's lap? And have you ever noticed that young children, when they are very upset, tend to rock back and forth to comfort themselves? This instinctive behavior serves a real purpose. Rhythmic rocking helps to counteract the panic messages being sent to the brain; it also provides a gentle massage to your stressed-out internal organs. Rocking encourages your brain to ignore many of the panic messages it is getting and slowly your levels of stress will begin to drop. Many office chairs now come with a rocking mechanism and in the home a rocking chair can become a family favorite to help deal with everything from crying infants to stressed-out executives.

TRY MEDITATION

Meditation is a good way to let go of your worries for a short period of time. You can meditate anywhere. Often meditation involves deep regular breathing, which in itself is relaxing.

In meditation, the idea is to empty your mind. When you

do this, you leave your worries behind, making space for more positive, relaxing thoughts. Some would argue, perhaps rightly, that emptying your mind can be difficult to do in a busy office or on a crowded train. This will be true at first. However, the more you practice, the more you will be able to take a five-minute meditation break wherever you are.

If your mind isn't completely empty as you begin to meditate, don't worry. Some people take on meditation as if it were just another stressful job. They become very critical of themselves if a persistent thought comes into their heads while they are supposed to be meditating, or if they can only hold onto emptiness for so long before they start to worry about some aspect of their lives.

If this happens to you, don't be too hard on yourself. The best way to deal with intrusive thoughts during meditation is to acknowledge them rather than fight them. Some people do this in a nonjudgmental way by saying "thinking" to themselves each time a new thought pops up and then letting the thought go. After a while, it will become easier to have a meditation break in which thoughts don't come intruding into your rest time.

GUIDED IMAGERY

Our bodies react to thoughts and images, which is why one aspect of meditation, known as guided imagery, may be useful. Guided imagery is a flow of thoughts that you can see, hear, feel, smell, or even taste in your imagination. It is legitimate daydreaming for adults.

We all engage in guided imagery from time to time probably without knowing it. Perhaps the best example of guided imagery in our everyday lives is worry. When we worry about something we allow ourselves to imagine a whole series of "what ifs." We follow pictures in our minds of the many possibilities, we check out our emotional responses to each situation, we may even be aware of how our bodies respond, with churning stomachs and racing hearts, as we run through these scenarios. If you have ever done this and made yourself feel worse, you have the ability to do this and make yourself feel better. Worrying yourself sick and imagining yourself well are two sides of the same coin.

A useful guided image when you have a headache is to imagine you are somewhere warm, that your muscles are like ice cubes melting in the warm sun. As the sun penetrates deeper and deeper, reaching every muscle, the tension just melts away, leaving you relaxed and refreshed.

Another good trick is to personify your headache—to imagine it a person or creature. All body symptoms have a message. If you are not particularly good at listening to the language of the body, imagine that it can talk to you in your language. During your guided imagery, make a note of who the character is, what it looks like, what it has to say to you, and what you have to say to it. A great deal of useful information can be gained from this deceptively simple exercise.

Of course, you don't have to follow any prescribed guided image if you don't want to. Any image that makes you feel better will do. It can be equally effective to meditate upon a happy, restful, or relaxing memory or make up a fantasy of where you would like to be now or whom you would like to be with.

MASSAGE

Even short massages can relieve tension. Many practitioners will come to your workplace and provide short, on-site massage.

This is a sound investment in employee health. In one study from the United States, the effectiveness of a fifteen-minute on-site massage on reducing stress was measured. Researchers found that after receiving such a massage, individuals experienced significantly lowered blood pressure.

Tension at work, whether from deadlines or uncomfortable chairs, can contribute to headaches in the workplace. If you and your colleagues are experiencing more than your fair share of headaches, perhaps it's time to arrange for a masseuse or aromatherapist to pay weekly visits. A short massage break will do you infinitely more good than a coffee or cigarette break.

TAKE A WALK

If you are under a lot of pressure, it is particularly important to get regular exercise, as this will help you let off steam and counterbalance the effects of stress. Exercise has been shown in many studies to help reduce stress levels. If you are at work and cannot simply pop out to the gym, make sure that you have enough time to go out, take a walk, and get some fresh air. In the summer, you can find a secluded spot and eat your lunch outside.

GET A (SPIRITUAL) LIFE

For some people, headache is a sign of emptiness. Studies have shown that a commitment to your own spirituality can reduce stress. Meditation is primarily practiced by those people who don't pray. The effect of prayer on the body is the same as meditation—it takes people out of themselves and allows them to place their faith in something bigger than their day-to-day experiences. There are many studies proving that people who engage in spiritual practices live healthier and longer lives. People who are involved in organized religions may be encouraged by their faith to take better all-round care of themselves. They are more able to let go of the belief that life "should" be more perfect than it is. Also, they can release some of their daily burdens to whichever higher being they acknowledge.

CHAPTER 5

The Food Factor

FOOD AS A TRIGGER

If food gives you a headache, probably you are intolerant or allergic to it or to the ingredients contained in it. Experts now agree that food sensitivity is an important cause of headaches. However, there continues to be confusion over which foods are involved.

Some experts believe wheat, corn, milk, sugars, and oranges are the culprits. Others speculate that foods containing amines—which cause the blood vessels to contract—are the main cause. Still others suggest that foods with a high copper content—chocolate, nuts, shellfish, and wheat germ—may trigger migraine. In truth, there is overlap between potential triggers. For instance, chocolate contains sugar, caffeine, and amines. Citrus can increase copper absorption, and the food additive MSG binds to citrus and transports it around the body. Not surprisingly, both citrus and MSG are also linked to migraine headaches. None of these foods, in themselves, is bad. But certain foods have been repeatedly implicated in recurrent headaches. The fact is that anyone can be sensitive to almost anything and food intolerance and allergy—like headaches—can be highly individual.

When you eat a food which you are allergic or intolerant to, your body reacts as if it had been poisoned. Symptoms can include nausea, stomach pains, fatigue, and headaches. There now seems to be little doubt that food sensitivity is a major contributing factor to migraine headaches (see the table on pages 47-48). But a migraine reaction is just the extreme end of a spectrum of reactions which may also include tension-like headaches (since the body will be under stress each time you ingest a food that it cannot tolerate). Many carefully conducted studies have shown that when the offending food is removed from an individual's diet, headaches and their accompanying symptoms tend to disappear as well.

Take, for example, one famous study at a London hospital in 1983. More than ninety percent of children who had severe, frequent migraines recovered once the foods they were allergic to were omitted from their diets. The results were unequivocal and produced a rate of cure which no medication can match.

There is no clear understanding of how many people will benefit from removing potential allergens from their diet. Research puts the numbers at anywhere from thirty to ninety percent. We do know that all types of headaches are successfully treated by this action.

There are several methods which you can use to detect a food allergy. You can opt for a blood test which will look for specific antigens (chemicals produced by your body as a reaction to the allergic components in specific foods). Many people feel that this is the most accurate way to detect food allergies. However, the accuracy of the results will depend on the laboratory.

FOODS MOST LIKELY TO CAUSE MIGRAINE

In the textbook *The Encyclopaedia of Natural Medicine*, considered by many to be the standard reference for natural remedies, authors Michael Murray and Joseph Pizzorno review three studies of food as a migraine trigger. This table is a summary of their findings. The percentages represent the range of individuals whose headaches were triggered by that food. Bear in mind that each individual can have more than one trigger.

Food	Percentage
Cow's milk	57–67%
Wheat	43–57%
Chocolate	26–57%
Egg	22 60%
Orange	13–52%
Cheese	32%
Tomato	14–32%
Rye	30%
Rice	30%
Fish (incl. shellfish)	17–29%
Grapes	12–33%
Onion	24%
Soy	17–24%
Pork	17–22%
Peanuts	12–29%
Alcohol	9–29%
Walnuts	19%
Beef	14–20%
Tea	17%
Coffee	15–19%

Food	Percentage
Nuts	12–19%
Goat's milk	14–15%
Oats	15%
Cane sugar	7–19%
Yeast	12–14%
Apple	12%
Peach	12%
Potato	12%
Chicken	7–14%
Banana	4–7%
Strawberry	7%
Melon	7%
Carrot	7%

An equally effective way of gauging whether a particular food disagrees with you is to simply remove it from your diet, along with other likely culprits, for a month or two. Then, reintroduce them one at a time, monitoring carefully how your body reacts. It is particularly important to do it this way, because reactions to foods are not always immediate. It can take twenty minutes to eight hours or more to produce a reaction.

While you are removing foods from your diet, be especially mindful of those foods you really crave—these are probably the foods that you are most sensitive to. If you are considering removing a wide range of foods all at once, you should consider seeking the guidance of a qualified nutritionist. You do not want to run the risk of becoming run-down or undernourished in the process.

OTHER TRIGGERS

There are other dietary factors that you should also consider. Most are common in processed convenience foods. Some, for example, specific food ingredients and additives, such as the orange color tartrazine, benzoic acid, monosodium glutamate (MSG), and the nitrates used to preserve meats, will be listed on the labels of processed foods. Others, such as those labeled as "flavorings" and "aromas," are more vague. These can be made up of literally hundreds of synthetic chemicals. Manufacturers are not obliged to list them on their packaging. You will never really know which of these chemicals is hurting you. While governments and regulatory bodies claim that food additives are safe, nutritionists believe otherwise. One of the best ways to eliminate potential allergens of this type is to eat only fresh foods. Processed foods contain too much chemical junk and even if you are not allergic or intolerant to it, it will certainly hurt your body.

ALCOHOL

Alcohol is cited often by migraine sufferers as a trigger. It is probably not the alcohol itself that gives you a headache, so don't bother switching to a low-alcohol brew. Some wines and beers contain unpleasant chemicals and preservatives, particularly sulfites, which many people are sensitive to. If you are not sulfite sensitive, but wine still gives you a headache, try switching to organic wines, which will not have the pesticide content of regular wines.

AMINES

These naturally occurring substances are strongly linked to headaches of all types. Amines can trigger a chemical process that causes the bloodstream to be flooded with serotonin, causing the blood vessels to contract. Individuals who are prone to migraines are particularly sensitive to amines, and may even have low levels of a special enzyme which normally breaks down the amines in food.

Any fermented, pickled, or marinated food will be high in amines. Other foods containing high levels of amines include avocados, bananas, cabbage, eggplant, pineapple, plums, potatoes, canned fish, caffeinated drinks, chicken liver, MSG, chocolate, citrus fruits, nuts, processed meats, raisins, ripened cheese, aged meats, yeast extracts, sourdough bread, onions, and lentils. Red wine contains tyramine and should be avoided by those who suffer from chronic headaches, especially migraine sufferers.

ARTIFICIAL SWEETENERS

People who use products sweetened with aspartame may be putting themselves at risk for chronic headaches. In one study at the University of Florida, the incidence of migraine doubled in participants exposed to aspartame. Airline pilots who consume large amounts of diet sodas in order to stave off dehydration on long-distance flights experience more headaches than those who don't.

Aspartame is an excitotoxin—it is one of a number of chemicals that have been shown to damage the nervous system through overstimulation. There is accumulating evidence that this product, which contains the vasodilator phenylalanine, may be a factor in tension and migraine headaches. In one study, more than eight percent of migraine sufferers found their symptoms were triggered by aspartame. Aspartame is found in nearly all commercially produced sweetened foods such as sodas, fruit drinks, yogurts, chewing gums, ready-made and packaged desserts, candy, ice-cream cakes, cookies, and even some multi-vitamins. If a product claims to have "no added sugar," it is probably sweetened with aspartame.

CAFFEINE

Caffeine dilates the blood vessels. Studies show that men and women who consume four to five cups of coffee or black tea daily are more likely to suffer from headaches. Be aware that if you choose to reduce or cut out coffee and tea altogether, you may experience a short period where your headaches get worse. Caffeine withdrawal—just like analgesic withdrawal—can cause rebound headaches. You may also experience some drowsiness and fatigue as well as tremors. These symptoms will pass and in a short while you will begin to feel more energy and less of a tendency toward headaches.

Note also that decaffeinated coffee or tea is not always a solution—for some it can cause an increase in headaches. Conventionally decaffeinated coffee and tea contain harsh chemicals which may trigger headaches and are certainly not healthy. If you want to try and make the switch to a decaffeinated brew, make sure it is a product in which the caffeine has been removed by a water filtration method and not by a chemical process.

Going cold turkey may be your best hope if you are trying to give up caffeine. Try substituting herbal teas or cereal drinks made from roasted chicory or barley. Your taste buds will soon adapt. In the meantime, watch out for hidden sources of caffeine such as sodas and chocolate.

CHOCOLATE

Reactions to chocolate are probably due to its high amine content, in particular the chemicals phenylethylamine and tyramine. Both phenylethylamine and tyramine act on the blood vessels. Perhaps the best way to test your reaction to chocolate is to abstain for a week or two and then reintroduce it into your diet. If your symptoms get worse, you will have proof that chocolate should be eliminated from your diet.

CURED MEATS

If sausages, bacon, hot dogs, and deli meats give you a headache it is probably because of the nitrates and nitrites used as preservatives. Although there is ample evidence that nitrates and nitrites can cause illness and may even be carcinogenic, no moves have been made to outlaw them. The characteristic flavor of bacon is impossible without them. The only solution is to avoid nitrates by avoiding the foods which contain them.

DAIRY PRODUCTS

Milk is a common headache trigger. Some people may be intolerant to milk in general. Cheese (particularly aged cheese) contains the amines phenylethylamine and tyramine, and so does sour cream. The lactase content of milk may be the culprit in some headaches.

MONOSODIUM GLUTAMATE (MSG)

Monosodium glutamate is widely used in processed foods to make them taste better than they would otherwise. Like aspartame, it is an excitotoxin. A number of headache sufferers report MSG as a trigger. There is accumulating evidence that this chemical wreaks havoc in the body in other ways. In studies where rats were given MSG in doses equivalent to that in baby food, they developed brain lesions and other disturbing symptoms.

MSG is found in nearly all processed foods, including potato chips, packaged soups, ready-made meals, meat tenderizers, and canned meats. It goes by many names including natural flavorings, hydrolyzed vegetable protein (HVP), kombu extract, hydrolyzed plant protein (HPP), calcium caseinate, autolyzed yeast, and sodium caseinate.

PESTICIDES

Other potential allergens in food are the pesticides and fungicides used during their growth, transport, storage, and display in supermarkets. Few people realize, for instance, that apples may be stored for six months or more before they go on display. All the while they will be sprayed with chemicals to keep them looking fresh. In supermarkets today you can find arsenic on your strawberries, DDT on your spinach, paraffin on your cucumbers and peppers, and bananas ripened with ethylene gas.

The range of potentially harmful chemicals you can ingest is simply vast. If a number of otherwise unrelated produce items seem to give you a headache, it may not be the food but the pesticide residue that is the problem. Washing won't help remove it all, since pesticide residue is remarkably stubborn. The best way to test if you are allergic to pesticides is to switch to organic produce and see if it produces the same effect.

THE HIGH-CARBOHYDRATE DIET

Doctors and nutritionists are always telling us that a diet high in carbohydrates is healthy. For headache sufferers this is particularly true. A diet based on complex carbohydrates, such as whole grains, beans, peas, and other seed foods, has been shown to increase the amount of the amino acid tryptophan available in the body. Tryptophan is converted in the body into serotonin, which helps regulate the diameter of blood vessels and enhances our feeling of well-being.

A high-carbohydrate diet can also reduce migraines caused by low blood sugar. Unrefined carbohydrates and strict avoidance of sugars can minimize people's up and down swings in blood sugar, which may be effective in reducing the duration and severity of migraines. If you get headaches when you haven't eaten for a few hours, it might be a good idea to ask your doctor to test for hypoglycemia.

If you suspect hypoglycemia, try eating small meals throughout the day. Don't binge on chocolate and other empty snacks. Instead, make sure you have a steady supply of whole foods such as fruits, vegetables, and nuts on hand. Apple juice will release sugar more slowly into your bloodstream than other juices. Think also about how you start your day. Highly processed cereals such as corn flakes may not be the best choice. These cereals are usually boiled, then baked, and are probably closer to being a simple sugar (which will sharply elevate your blood sugar and then just as sharply drop it) than the complex carbohydrates found in oatmeal and muesli, which will keep your blood sugar even over a longer period of time.

As with all dietary advice, there are exceptions and some people do worse on a high-carbohydrate diet.

Just to confuse matters, a low-carbohydrate diet has also been advocated as a headache treatment. This diet is probably most appropriate when headaches are a symptom of high levels of sugar in the blood. As the sugar is metabolized, it can cause a type of rebound hypoglycemia. Both the low-carbohydrate diet and a low-sugar diet have been successful in treating this type of headache.

HELPFUL SUPPLEMENTS

Supplements can never replace a good diet, but for some people, taking extra amounts of vitamin B6, magnesium, lithium, and/or essential fatty acids may help relieve migraine symptoms.

People who are particularly prone to migraine may be low in magnesium. Studies of women suggest that migraine symptoms improve once a magnesium deficiency has been identified and corrected. It is best to combine B6 with your magnesium supplement to enhance its effectiveness.

The whole B-complex will be useful if you are under a lot of stress, but you might want to consider upping your intake of B2 (riboflavin) if you suffer from regular migraines. In a recent study, participants who reported between two and eight migraine attacks per month took a relatively high dose of B2 (400 mg) each day, and started to experience improvement after just two months. It was speculated that B2 helps build up the body's energy reserves—which can be depleted by recurring migraine attacks—making recovery more swift. Although riboflavin appears to be safe in daily doses up to 600 mg, you may not wish to take this much B2 without the guidance of a qualified nutritionist. However, you can confidently take a good-quality B-complex which contains around 100 mg of each of the B vitamins.

You should also try to include more essential fatty acids in your diet. Fatty acids are divided into two main groups: the

Omega 6 group, which comes from such sources as evening primrose oil, borage oil, and black currant seed oil; and the Omega 3 family, which comes from oily fish, flax seeds, and pumpkin seeds. We need both for good health, usually taken in a ratio of 2:1, Omega 6 to Omega 3.

Boosting the intake of the Omega 3 family in particular has been shown to be beneficial in headache sufferers. There have been studies showing that patients who have a severe migraine, and who do not respond to conventional treatment, often respond to supplements of fish oils. You can up your intake with any number of good quality supplements on the market. However, the best and most flavorful way to do this is to increase your consumption of oily fish such as salmon, herring, and mackerel as well as increasing seed foods such as linseed, pumpkin, sunflower, and flax seeds, all of which are delicious as a topping on salads and cereals.

If you must take supplements, those which contain fish oils may be particularly useful. However, there has been concern among nutritionists that some fish oils may be contaminated with mercury. If this is also a concern for you, you should take supplements which source their Omega 3 fatty acids from linseed, flax, and other seeds which are equally as good. Try taking 1000 mg (or the equivalent of around 50–100 mg Omega 3) of fish or seed-based oil daily for six weeks—you may find that it reduces both the frequency and severity of your migraine symptoms.

EXPANSION AND CONTRACTION

If all the information on food and headaches presented so far seems a bit daunting, consider the system worked out by Annemarie Colbin, American nutritionist and founder of the

Institute of Food and Health in New York. Ms. Colbin believes that headaches are a sign of systemic imbalance. She classifies food-related headaches either as expansion or contraction headaches, with side categories for "liver" headaches, caffeine withdrawal headaches, and others. Her system is based on the ancient Chinese belief that certain foods are expansive and others are contractive, and that an imbalance of these foods in the diet causes imbalance in the body.

Expansion headaches, according to Colbin's system, are usually the result of too much liquid of any kind, including fruit juice, alcohol, ice cream, and other cold and highly sugared foods. These headaches can, she says, be remedied in two to fifteen minutes by eating salty, contractive foods which counterbalance the effect. You might try the following:

- Gomasio (sesame salt): You can make this by grinding up one cup of raw sesame seeds. Add to the half-crushed mixture two teaspoons of salt, then grind well into the seed mixture.
- Umeboshi plums: You can buy these Japanese pickled plums in most health food shops. They taste salty-sour. The best brands have no ingredients other than plums, salt, water, and maybe beefsteak (chiso) leaves. Alternatively, you can buy paste made from umeboshi that you can take a fingerful of when you have an expansive headache.
- Just a few brine-made olives may also help to ease your headache pain.

Contraction headaches are usually the result of:
- Tension
- Overwork
- Heat

- Meats and salty foods (especially taken on an empty stomach)
- Lack of food and/or fluids
- Excess mental concentration or physical activity in addition to the above

These headaches can take a little longer to alleviate in some cases, but the following remedies should work within five minutes to twenty-four hours. They consist of something cool and liquid, sweet, or sour, such as:

- Apple or apricot juice: Make sure it is the best quality you can afford, preferably fresh pressed and if possible organic.
- Cold unsweetened applesauce (or other cooked fruit).

In Ms. Colbin's system, migraines are known as liver headaches, usually occurring two, four, or even eight hours after eating a food which unbalances the system. This is why it can be so difficult to link to the offending food. In her experience, these headaches are usually the result of eating fatty foods on an empty stomach, including fried eggs or cheese for breakfast, and salads with oily dressings and avocado. To remedy this type of headache, use the same remedies as for contraction headaches. In addition, try lemon tea.

This remedy can be made at home from the following ingredients. Make one cup of lemon tea (hot water with the juice of half a lemon). Add a tablespoon of maple syrup (you can add more to taste if you prefer). Next, add a pinch of cayenne pepper or five drops of Tabasco sauce (these have a cooling effect) or 2 teaspoons of fresh grated ginger (this has a warming effect)—be guided by your inclinations. Stir well and drink hot.

Caffeine withdrawal headaches should be treated as

contraction headaches. If you are not sure which type of headache you have, you can find out relatively quickly by having a tiny bite of umeboshi plum, or a fingerful of plum paste. If you remain the same or get better, you have an expansive headache; if you get worse, you have a contractive or liver headache.

CHAPTER 6

Is Your Home Giving You a Headache?

Your home should be a haven where you can rest and your body can repair itself. Unfortunately, many of our homes are not safe. In fact, indoor pollution is now recognized as more of a threat to our health than outdoor pollution. The cleaning supplies we use in our kitchens and bathrooms—the very ones which promise to make our homes healthier by removing "harmful bacteria"; the pesticides we use on our lawns; the fumes we inhale while cooking or heating our homes; the volatile chemicals emitted from aerosol sprays, carpets, and plastics; and the electromagnetic field (EMF) emitted from all our household appliances can all cause chronic health problems.

Indoor air pollution has become a considerable problem in recent decades. Lance Wallace, an environmental expert working for the Environmental Protection Agency (EPA), conducted a survey of 600 homes in six cities and found that concentrations of twenty toxic or carcinogenic (cancer-causing) chemicals were up to fifty times higher indoors than outdoors.

Many of the chemicals used in household products are highly volatile—they evaporate easily and can be inhaled. Others, sprayed from aerosol cans or hand pumps, release a shower of microscopic, easily inhaled particles known as volatile organic chemicals, or VOCs.

You are highly likely to be exposed to harmful chemicals while you are showering, washing dishes, and flushing the toilet. Many industrial solvents and contaminants such as benzene and methylene chloride get dumped into our water supply and can easily pass through the skin into the body during showers, baths, and dishwashing. More importantly, these chemicals become gases at room temperature and are then easily inhaled. According to at least two environmental studies, the amount of industrial VOCs inhaled during a fifteen-minute shower with contaminated water is equivalent to drinking about eight glasses of contaminated water. The longer and hotter the shower, the more chemicals build up in the air. Baths also produce this effect, but to a much smaller extent.

Here is what you can do to avoid inhaling chemicals in your home. Avoid using all aerosols, no matter what propellant is used. Every time you use an aerosol can you will inhale high concentrations of its contents.

Some headache sufferers are very sensitive to dust, but there is another good reason to keep dust levels as low as you can in your house. Dust particles absorb VOCs and increase their concentration in the air. Limit the time you spend in the shower and make sure the water is warm to cool and finish off with a cool to cold rinse. When you shower, open a window to let waterborne chemicals out and close the bathroom door to prevent them from getting to other areas of the house.

There is now substantial scientific data to suggest that carpeting may be bad for your health. Although many of us believe that we have made great progress since the days of bare wood floors, carpets are constantly giving off dangerous gases.

Although we have long known this about new carpets, research suggests that even older carpets may still be emitting chemicals which can cause illness. Writing in *The Journal of Nutritional and Environmental Medicine*, Rosalind Anderson reported that she analyzed one hundred and twenty-five carpet samples ranging from one week to twelve years old. She put them in the cages containing mice and found that the mice's breathing rate was immediately decreased. Their faces became swollen, their posture was altered, they became hyperactive, and they lost their balance. Even convulsions and death followed. She identified over two hundred different toxic chemicals being given off by modern carpets. In humans, common reactions include flu-like symptoms, muscle pain, headache, fatigue, tremors, memory loss, and diminished ability to concentrate. Carpets are also very efficient at trapping outdoor pollutants, partly because we track these pollutants in from the garden and other places, and because we use pesticides indoors. The No-Pest strips which we hang on walls and from light fixtures contain the cancer-causing insecticide dichlorvos (DDVP). In America, an EPA report on non-occupational pesticide exposure identified at least five pesticides at levels up to ten times greater indoors than outdoors.

If you are headachy and ill at home, maybe it's time to consider bare wood flooring. To protect yourself and your family from pesticides and other pollutants, take your shoes off before entering the house. Pesticides should be used sparingly, if at all. Moreover, you should use only enough of the product to get the job done. Read the labels and look for chemicals such as chlordane, and heptachlor, commonly used in garden insecticides, moth and termite proofing, as well as for other purposes.

Better yet, try using some of the organic pesticides now on the market.

HEAVY METAL

Metal toxicity can cause agonizing headaches in some individuals. It's all around us. For instance, if you have a mouth full of fillings, it is likely that mercury is slowly leaking into your system. Mercury-sensitive individuals will suffer a range of health problems such as allergies, fatigue, dizziness, headaches, nausea, and chronic fatigue.

The quality of the tap water we drink is often pretty poor. Filtration processes don't always remove nitrates and other chemical poisons. Also, our water contains many heavy metals, including aluminum and chlorine—both of which are added to some types of water at treatment plants—and lead. Aluminum has been associated with neurological problems such as Alzheimer's disease, and chloride has been associated with damage to the blood vessels and anemia. Lead is another major metal pollutant and it is all around us. It is a neurotoxin—it can damage the brain and nervous system. In studies on children, lead has been shown to impede their intellectual growth. The main source of lead poisoning in one study in Edinburgh, commissioned by Britain's Medical Research Council, was water. Lead exposure can also cause high blood pressure—a contributing factor in headaches. While water is a main source of lead, we can also inhale it from car emissions.

To avoid heavy metal poisoning, consider switching to bottled water, or a water filtration system. If you wish to go on using tap water, make sure you run the tap for at least two minutes before using the water for cooking or drinking. If you suspect mercury poisoning from fillings, you can get tested and, if necessary, have your mercury fillings removed.

Don't use enameled cookware—a major source of the toxic metal cadmium. Cadmium poisoning has been linked to a wide range of disorders, including chronic headaches. It is also a well-known carcinogen. Other common sources of cadmium are cigarette smoke and excessive tea and coffee drinking.

ELECTRICAL SENSITIVITY

Electrical sensitivity is an environmentally triggered illness with symptoms similar to chemical sensitivity. It is just beginning to be recognized by some doctors and scientists. Throughout our homes and in our offices, we have a number of electrically powered devices which are intended to make our lives easier. It's hard to imagine that these gadgets might produce side effects which could cause headaches and other health problems. Nevertheless, exposure to electromagnetic fields (EMFs) from power lines, computers, and motors affect the nervous system, causing symptoms not unlike chronic fatigue.

In a recent survey published by the magazine *Electrical Sensitivity*, headache was among the most common symptoms experienced by those suffering from electrical sensitivity. Other symptoms included fatigue and weakness, skin rashes, confusion, and poor concentration.

Airborne particles including water, dust, and toxic chemicals concentrate close to electric fields. One study in Norway, for instance, showed that they tend to concentrate under power lines and concluded that airborne products are attracted to sources of power. Researchers are now turning their attention to the question of whether other airborne toxins such as bacteria might also be concentrated around electric fields, increasing toxic potential. To limit the effect of EMFs in your home, try repositioning your furniture. Avoid locating beds or chairs too close to significant domestic sources of EMFs such as electricity meters or TVs. Allow at least six to eight feet from such sources, especially for beds. Bedside radio alarms, whether electric or battery powered, should be at least two feet from your head. Don't plug appliances in near your bed and don't use an electric blanket; if you do, switch it off, or better yet unplug it, before going to bed. Remember that electrical fields can be generated even by appliances that are switched off.

In addition to EMFs, computers, laser printers, copiers, and fax machines release volatile organic chemicals into the air when they operate. Where possible, keep the air clean by opening your window when using these machines, or have an exhaust fan or air purifier that contains a charcoal filter (other types do not remove chemicals) installed nearby.

PLASTIC FANTASTIC?

Many common household products emit chemicals. Because of the extensive use of building materials and furnishings that release formaldehyde, exposure to it is almost inescapable in modern indoor environments. The greatest levels are given off by the glue that holds together particle board and plywood paneling. The brightly colored plastics which are now used for everything from storage to cleaning and kitchen implements, from waste paper bins to the casings on our electrical equipment, emit formaldehyde. So do new carpets, no-iron clothes, upholstery, foam insulation, latex paint, space heaters, new paper, and some cosmetics such as shampoo, nail polish, skin creams, and hair sprays.

Although formaldehyde emission decreases with time, high

humidity or moisture can increase its release from particle board and paneling. Chronic exposure to formaldehyde has been shown to produce a number of unpleasant symptoms including headaches, memory loss, drowsiness, nausea, dizziness, shortness of breath, irritation of the eyes and nose, and even cancer.

THE TOXIC BEAUTY TRAP

If you suffer from headaches regularly, you may be a victim of the toxic beauty trap. There are several things you can watch out for and eliminate. Any product with bright colors (striped toothpaste, colored mouthwash, shampoo, deodorant, etc.) should be used with caution, since many of these contain synthetic dyes which have been implicated in a number of health problems. Perfumed products should also be regarded with suspicion.

If you suspect that chemical sensitivity is a trigger in your headaches, it's time to make the switch to cosmetics that are not colored or perfumed. Remember, neither the color of the product nor its scent add to its effectiveness. Don't be fooled by products that say they are natural—the word is highly abused and overused in the cosmetic and toiletry industry. Usually it means that synthetic petrochemicals have been used to approximate the real thing. For instance, if a product label says it contains the natural smell of lemons, this does not mean that they have used lemon essential oils to enhance its scent. It is more likely to be a synthetic version made up of literally hundreds of different chemicals. Unless a product lists the proper Latin name for essential oils, they are not using them as a scent.

A FINAL WORD

It is not possible to protect ourselves from every potential irritant in the environment. This is the world we have built and we have to live in it. Nevertheless, if you do suffer from chronic health problems, it is important to try to reduce the total load on your body. It will certainly improve your overall health. For some individuals, it may signal the end of a headache pain which has been plaguing them for years.

CHAPTER 7

Herbal Remedies

While herbal remedies still conjure up images of witches' brew to some people, there is much scientific validation for their use. Herbs have long been an essential part of medicine, and many of today's synthetic medicines have been copied (not always successfully) from herbal "blueprints." According to the World Health Organization, herbal medicine is the third most widely used type of medicine in the world. It is also one of the oldest forms of medicine.

When paleontologists discovered many herb fossils at ancient dwelling sites, it confirmed a long-held suspicion that medicinal herbs have been in use almost as long as man has been walking the Earth. The uses of herbs have been passed down from generation to generation as part of an oral tradition, long before we began to use books to record such information. Ancient Eastern civilizations used many animal, plant, and mineral remedies. Hippocrates knew and used herbs grown near where he lived. Herbal remedies continued to be used throughout Roman times. The Persians and Arabs added new remedies of their own.

Even as late as the early nineteenth century, physicians were still receiving stiff competition from traditional healers. In

America, the early settlers got valuable information about the healing power of native herbs from the natives. By the late 1800s, however, the scientific community began to isolate the active ingredients in many natural substances so that they could eventually be synthesized in the laboratory. It wasn't long before they were. But it is questionable whether synthesized products are as valuable as the originals.

Herbal remedies can be used alone or to complement conventional care. There are herbs to treat specific conditions, to ease pain and inflammation, relax or stimulate organs, fight bacteria, and boost the immune system. Herbs can be used in many different forms: capsules and tablets made from the dried or powdered plant; extracts where the juice has been squeezed from the fresh plant; tinctures where the plant has been steeped in alcohol, vinegar, or glycerin; or teas which can be made from both the dried and fresh leaves, flowers, root, and bark of the plant. Generally speaking, the less processing that has gone into the preparation of the remedy, the more you will benefit from it. This is why some herbalists recommend extracts and tinctures as the most effective way to take herbs. Herbal remedies can be taken internally and applied externally as ointments, creams, and essential oils.

Herbs are powerful medicine and should be taken with the same caution and respect that you would take any medication. You should certainly ask questions: What is the herb? Is it from an organic source? What effect will it have on me? Are there any side effects I should watch out for? Does it have any adverse interactions with conventional medications?

HERBS FOR HEADACHES

Herbs can boost the body's own ability to fight off infection—

useful if your headache has a viral origin. They can detoxify the body and so can help in cases of toxic build-up. Herbs can be used to help rebalance hormones safely and can relieve pain.

Whatever type of herb you use, it is important to understand that herbs act more slowly than conventional medicine. The aim is to build health from the inside out and this can take time, particularly if your health has been poor for some years. Several herbs have shown promise in research done on headache sufferers. Most of these herbs can be bought in over-the-counter preparations from your local health food store.

Capsaicin is the active ingredient found in cayenne pepper. It is one of the most widely used herbs for headache relief. It can be taken internally in small amounts, but it more often is applied as a cream to the site of the pain. When a cream containing capsaicin is applied to the skin, it blocks pain signals, and it diminishes the chemical transmitters that cause pain impulses. The best products are those which contain 0.025 to 0.075 percent standardized capsaicin. These are generally available in health food shops.

Cayenne has minimal side effects. In rare cases, people have reported allergic reactions including rashes. Taken internally, it sometimes can cause digestive tract inflammation. It appears that these side effects are most common at the beginning of treatment and that the body quickly builds up a tolerance to cayenne. If you are taking cayenne orally, the best way to avoid stomach upsets is to take it with food. Pregnant women should not use cayenne, as it can cause uterine contractions.

Feverfew is one of the most valuable herbs in the treatment of migraine. More than fifty scientific papers have been published in the past fifteen years examining the efficacy of feverfew. In 1988, at University Hospital in Nottingham, England, seventy-two migraine sufferers were randomly given either one capsule containing dried feverfew leaves or a matching placebo for four months. The treatments were then switched, with the placebo group receiving feverfew and vice versa, for a further four months. In the feverfew group, the number of migraine attacks fell by twenty-four percent, and significantly fewer working days were lost to headache compared to the placebo group. The feverfew group also experienced a reduction in the number and severity of migraine attacks and the degree of vomiting. In another study, when migraine sufferers who regularly took the herb were unknowingly given a placebo instead, their migraines worsened.

Feverfew is best taken in tablet form since the dried leaves can be bitter and with tea there is no way of guaranteeing a consistent strength. The active ingredient in the herb is thought to be parthenolide, although a recent analysis of studies at the University of Exeter suggests that there may be other beneficial, but as yet unidentified, ingredients in the whole plant.

However, consumers beware. When researchers in Nottingham tested several dried preparations, they found parthenolide levels varied widely between products and could not be detected at all in some. Make sure you check the label of any preparation you buy. It should contain at least 0.2 percent of parthenolide in every 125 mg of feverfew leaf powder to be effective.

Feverfew is generally free from side effects. However, certain restrictions do apply. Children under two should not be given feverfew, and pregnant women should also avoid it, since it can cause miscarriage.

White Willow Bark is probably the original non-steroid, anti-inflammatory drug (NSAID). It has been used as a pain reliever since 500 B.C. By the eighteenth century, European healers were employing it to treat fevers. The active ingredient of white willow bark (Salix alba) is salicin, which was isolated in 1828. When digested, this chemical is believed to be converted into salicylic acid—the same compound used in aspirin.

What makes this herb more appealing than aspirin, however, is that it has been shown to cause less gastrointestinal irritation. Headache sufferers who can't take aspirin because it upsets their stomachs may find that white willow bark, with its lower concentration of salicytes, is more acceptable. The downside is that it will not work as quickly as aspirin. But some other species of willow including *Salix daphnoids, Salix fragilis,* and *Salix purpurea,* contain higher concentrations of salicin. Look for these Latin names on any herbal pain reliever you buy.

While white willow bark is generally free from side effects, some people experience gastrointestinal upsets if they take too much of it regularly. Pregnant and nursing women should not use it, since salicin can increase the risk of birth defects. It should not be given to children under two, or to young children with colds, flu, or chicken pox, since like aspirin it has the potential to cause the sometimes fatal disease, Reyes' syndrome.

Ginger is commonly used in East Africa to treat a wide range of different headaches. Although ginger probably does not act directly on headaches, it can be particularly helpful in migraines where nausea and vomiting are present. If your headache is accompanied by stress and fatigue, ginger may perk you up (without the side effects of other stimulants such as caffeine), and thus relieve or diminish headache pain. Fresh ginger root is widely available in supermarkets and you can easily make a warming, reviving tea by grating it and pouring boiling water over it (1 teaspoon per cup). Using it liberally in your cooking will also be beneficial. It works equally well in sweet and savory dishes.

Garlic is another widely available remedy that may be beneficial for headache sufferers. First and foremost, garlic helps strengthen the immune system. It also reduces the stickiness of the blood, helping it to flow more freely. This is why it is often recommended for people with high blood pressure. Garlic has no known side effects, apart from garlic breath. If this worries you, you can always take it as an odorless or reduced odor capsule. For severe headaches, you may want to supplement with 1000 mg garlic oil capsules three times daily.

Valerian should be kept in your herbal medicine chest. It is one of the most potent herbal remedies for the relief of insomnia and has been shown to be at least as effective as benzodiazpines—but without the adverse effects. Valerian combines well with another sedative herb, passion flower, and many over-the-counter herbal remedies contain both. No adverse effects have been observed with valerian. However, be mindful that you do not need large doses to produce good results. Indeed, studies show that the quality of sleep is not improved with larger doses. In one study, 900 mg of valerian extract was no more powerful than 450 mg. Since it is obviously a powerful sedative, it is always best to take the minimum amount to produce restful sleep.

CHAPTER 8

Homeopathy

Homeopathy is one of the most gentle, yet most powerful alternatives available. It has never been shown to produce any adverse effect. An increasing number of people find it remarkably effective for the treatment of a wide range of disorders. Homeopathic treatment is based on the principle that like cures like. Thus, a remedy is prescribed that will produce the same symptoms in another normal person which the patient is currently suffering from. This is in complete contrast to conventional medicine, which traditionally treats a patient's symptoms with medicines that have the opposite effect. For example, in conventional medicine a patient suffering from constipation would be given something to loosen the bowels and someone suffering headache pain would be given medicines which block the pain.

In homeopathy, infinitesimal doses of medicines are derived from a variety of plant, mineral, chemical, and animal sources. These minute doses change and enhance the body's own capacity for both physical and emotional healing.

Homeopathy has been well researched and proven to work on a wide range of physical and emotional states. Homeopathy aims to treat the whole person; thus, individually chosen homeopathic remedies may help treat both the physical and emotional states that can trigger persistent and chronic headaches. Although many people report a swift and profound relief from their symptoms with homeopathy, most studies show that homeopathy tends to work slowly, but produces long-lasting results.

One of the reasons why homeopathy works so well for a large number of people is that treatment is based on the total symptom picture and the individual nature of the patient. Homeopathic evaluation is comprehensive and your practitioner will take a detailed personal history. Rather than suppressing symptoms, a homeopath will address the underlying cause. Because homeopathic remedies are safe and unlikely to produce side effects, they are appropriate for all groups, including the elderly and perhaps especially children.

Once a homeopathic practitioner has gathered your history, he or she will study your pattern of symptoms and choose a remedy best for you. You can do the same thing, albeit on a more limited scale. Your headache diary will help you to identify your major symptoms. It is particularly important if you are a beginner or are self-diagnosing to stick to major symptom patterns as the key to choosing a remedy. Compare your symptoms to those indicated for each remedy and try the one which most closely matches your own pattern.

If you select the wrong remedy, it simply won't work, and you will not suffer any unpleasant side effects. It is important if you buy homeopathic remedies over the counter not to use them as you would a conventional remedy. Often a single dose is all that is required. This is something which can be very difficult to understand if you have spent years taking medicine three or four times daily. If you are uncertain about how to take a remedy and the remedy's label is unclear, it is best to consult a qualified homeopathic therapist for advice.

Homeopathic remedies are available in a bafflingly wide range of doses from stores. However, the remedies which you can buy in most health food shops are commonly sold in two strengths, 6c and 30c (though occasionally the c is omitted on the label). The "c" means that one part of the remedy has been diluted with ninety-nine parts of water and alcohol. In a 6c remedy, for example, this process will have taken place six times. Less is more in homeopathy and although the 30c remedy has been diluted more times, it is considered more potent. Follow the dosage instruction on the label unless otherwise instructed. During a headache, try using one 6c tablet every half hour for occasional complaints, or one 30c tablet every half hour for more acute conditions. Stop taking the remedy at the first sign of improvement or after four hours, whichever comes first.

Homeopathic remedies are very delicate and certain things can antidote them. You should not take a remedy less than twenty minutes before or after food. Also avoid strong, highly flavored foods such as mints or cloves immediately before or after taking a remedy. While you are taking a homeopathic remedy, you should switch to a non-mint toothpaste—those flavored with fennel are a particularly good choice. You should not touch remedies with your bare hands. Always tip them straight from the lid of your storage bottle into your mouth. To make this easier, some commercially available remedies now come in single-dose dispensers. Remedies should always be stored in a cool dark place.

Scientists who do not believe that infinitesimal doses can work conclude that homeopathic cures are all in the mind. To test this theory, they compare the effect of homeopathic remedies against placebos—inert substances which are not thought to cause any reaction in the body. While studies into homeopathy have turned up mixed results, the general trend suggests that once the right remedy is selected, the patient experiences a reduction in the frequency, duration, and severity of headache pain. Mixed results in studies may be explained in part because researchers seldom allow for changing to a more suitable remedy should the first one fail to produce the desired results, as would happen in a genuine homeopathic consultation.

In one German study in 1991 which studied eight different remedies (singly or a combination of two), when compared with a placebo, homeopathy significantly reduced the number of headaches from ten attacks per month to 1.8 per month at the end of four months. This compared favorably to those individuals who were given a placebo; they experienced a much smaller reduction, from 9.9 per month to 7.9 per month.

When researchers at the Princess Margaret Migraine Clinic in London undertook a four-month trial of homeopathy in 1997, both groups improved (homeopathy nineteen percent, placebo sixteen percent). Eleven different homeopathic remedies were used in all. At first this seemed a disappointing result, but closer scrutiny revealed that the placebo worked best on the mild migraine attacks, while homeopathy seemed most effective on moderate to severe attacks. Most importantly, improvement in the placebo group began to be reversed after the fourth month, while slow improvement continued in the homeopathy group.

While almost any homeopathic remedy can help a headache, some are more commonly used than others. After looking at the ten most common remedies listed below, if you are still unsure which remedy is most suited to your symptom pattern, homeopath Dana Ullman recommends trying either Belladonna, Bryonia, or Nux Vomica, since these cover the most commonly experienced headache symptoms.

Belladonna is indicated for violent, throbbing, or drumming pain. This type of headache can cause extreme sensitivity and the least bit of light, noise, touch, strong or unusual smells, motion, or jarring brings on a new wave of pain. It can begin suddenly and may also go away suddenly. It may spread throughout the entire head or be localized in the forehead, where it may extend to the back of the head. Often the pupils are dilated and the face is flushed or feels hot, or there may be a high fever. Sometimes the hands and feet are cold. This type of headache, called The Belladonna Headache, characteristically strikes in the afternoon. Often the pain is made worse by climbing stairs, as well as going down a slope, escalator, or stairway. Hot sun will also aggravate the pain. Firm pressure to the head will often make the headache feel better, as will sitting down.

Bryonia is indicated when the headache is aggravated by motion. In fact, this is one of this headache's most important features. Even a slight motion of the eyes can make this headache worse. The pain can also be made worse by slight touch. It is generally worse in the morning. It may be felt immediately upon waking, but is just as likely to come on only after the person first moves in bed or gets out of bed. The pain is generally located in the forehead and extends to the back of the head, but is commonly centered over the left eye. It is experienced as a steady ache with very little throbbing. Sometimes there is a sense of fullness or heaviness in the head. During an attack, the head may also feel bruised. Nausea and vomiting and especially constipation may occur. You may feel irritable and irascible and want to be left alone. This headache generally gets better with firm pressure, rest, lying on the painful side, and cool drinks or compresses.

Gelsemium is a good remedy for headaches accompanied by muscle contractions. The pain is often right-sided and generally begins at the back of the head, often extending to the rest of the head or forehead. You may feel as though a band or hoop were bound tightly around your head. Or your head will feel full and swollen, and your face can be purple and congested looking. You may also feel dull, aching, and apathetic, with a weak, heavy feeling in your limbs. Your eyes may droop and you may look exhausted. Gelsemium is one of the few homeopathic remedies indicated for headaches preceded by a dimness of vision or the other visual disturbances so common in migraine attacks. The pain of this headache is not much affected by changes in room temperature, but other environmental factors such as light, noise, motion, and jarring do aggravate it. Napping, damp weather, tobacco smoke, and strong emotions will make the pain worse. Though not particularly irritable, you will want to be left alone. The pain is generally better if you move outdoors, put your head between your knees, take a walk, and drink stimulants such as coffee.

Natrum Mur is prescribed for the headache that is brought on by bright sunlight or prolonged periods of coughing. The pain can be blinding. It may feel as if your head is bursting or being pounded by a thousand tiny hammers. It is generally worse in the top of the head or over the eyes. Your face may lose all its color during an attack, which may last from sunrise to sunset. The pain may be worsened by prolonged mental effort, noise, or touch. You will not want to talk to or receive sympathy from others during an attack. What makes the pain feel better is cool, fresh air, or a cool bath, resting with your head elevated, being left alone, and skipping a meal.

Nux Vomica is prescribed for headaches brought on by overindulgence—food, drink, drugs, or staying up too late. These headaches can make you feel as if you have been beaten about the head. You may be irritable and feel sick and have a stomachache. You may have a bitter or sour taste in your mouth in the morning and queasiness, dizziness, nausea, or vomiting (dry heaves and gas are typical symptoms). The pain can be brought on by long periods of concentrated mental work. Cold air and wind will make it worse. This headache tends to be more prominent in the morning, particularly upon first waking, and tends to get better after the person is up and about. As with most headaches, motion may aggravate the symptoms, but shaking the head will be particularly painful. Lying on the painful side often makes the pain worse, and the sound of footsteps may be particularly irritating. Wrapping the head or being in a warm room may help to relieve the pain.

Phosphorous is a good remedy to use if your headaches are brought on by changes in atmospheric conditions, before a thunderstorm, for example. The headache can also be brought on by hunger, fright, or shock. The pain of a Phosphorous headache usually manifests as an aching over one eye. It is generally a throbbing, burning pain and can be accompanied by dizziness and vertigo. Being touched and lying on the painful side will make it worse, as will cold air and mental effort. These headaches tend to be worse in the morning and evening. Lying in a darkened room, massage, eating, a cool shower or bath, and a nap will often help improve symptoms.

Pulsatilla is a good remedy if your headaches often come on after meals, particularly if you have been eating warm or fatty foods. Nausea, digestive upset, and vomiting may also be a feature. Pulsatilla is good for those headaches which coincide with the menstrual cycle—before, during, and especially when the period ends—and also those that result from a frightening experience. The throbbing pain is most often felt in the forehead or on one side; however, it may change location frequently. Walking briskly may make the pain worse, whereas gentle motion, especially walking about slowly in the open air, may make the pain better. Pressure will also relieve the pain, but blowing the nose aggravates it. The Pulsatilla individual is emotionally mild and sensitive and may weep from the pain. Though a little irritable, the person is likely to want company and consolation.

Sanguinaria is for the headache that begins in the back of the head, but extends to and soon settles over the right eye or in the right side of the head. Right-sided headaches are covered by other remedies such as Gelsemium, but Sanguinaria is especially noted for this symptom. The pain is sharp, splitting, knife-like, and sometimes throbbing. Once again, nausea and vomiting occur at the height of the pain. Vomiting in particular may provide relief. Motion will make the pain worse, whereas sleep and firm pressure relieve it. This remedy suits headaches which occur in a consistent pattern, such as every seven days, and may be useful for cluster headaches or if you are having a classic migraine with visual-aura symptoms.

Sepia is for the headache that is usually connected with digestive symptoms. Often these headaches are brought on by skipping a meal. This headache can produce stinging, shooting pains over one eye—usually the left—accompanied by nausea and dizziness. In some cases, the roots of your hair will feel sensitive. The pain tends to strike in the late afternoons and evenings and is made worse by dampness, just before your period, by bending over, and by sex. You may also feel depressed and unable to cope. Vigorous exercise in fresh air can make the headache better, as will pressure and warm compresses on the painful points.

Sulphur is for the headache caused by low blood sugar. People who suffer from the Sulphur type of headache need to eat small, regular meals to combat hypoglycemia. The pain is somewhat different from the Sepia headache. You may feel dizzy and have a heavy, throbbing sensation in the crown of your head, or you may feel as if your brain was being squeezed. There may be pressure in the temples. This type of headache is made worse if you become overheated, especially while you are in bed and if you have exerted yourself too much. Alcohol will also make it worse. The headache tends to strike in mid-morning. It can also be brought on by sweet foods. Fresh air, particularly if the weather is warm and dry, movement, and walking all help to alleviate the pain.

CHAPTER 9

Acupuncture

Holistic practitioners and medical scientists agree on one thing: all life is made of energy. The Chinese call the life energy which surrounds and flows through us Qi, or Ch'i (pronounced *chee*). When this life force is disturbed, either because it is blocked or because it is moving too slowly or too fast, imbalance and illness will result. The Chinese believe that headaches are the result of blood stagnation and that stimulation of specific acupuncture points can help to relieve this stagnation.

The word acupuncture has two roots in Latin: *acus*, meaning needle and *punctura*, to puncture. In China thousands of years ago, a strange phenomenon was observed in times of war. Soldiers whose bodies were pierced by arrows sometimes recovered from illnesses which had plagued them for many years. Eventually, the notion evolved that, by penetrating the skin at certain points, diseases could be cured. Although acupuncture has been an important part of traditional Chinese medicine for more than 2,500 years, it is only over the last twenty years or so that it has come to be more widely accepted by healthcare practitioners and the general public in the West.

The World Health Organization has gone so far as to state that there is now sufficient medical evidence to support the effectiveness of acupuncture so that it may be considered an important part of primary health care. The usually conservative medical press is devoting more and more space to acupuncture. Recently, the *Journal of the American Medical Association* devoted an entire issue to alternative healthcare, which included a strong validation of acupuncture. The World Health Organization has gone even further by recommending that acupuncture be fully integrated into conventional medicine.

There are over 2,000 acupuncture points on the body, running along the twelve meridians, or energy channels. Each meridian is a biological pathway linked to a particular organ in the body; thus, each organ can be treated by stimulating the corresponding meridian. In everyday practice, however, only about 200 acupuncture points are commonly used. These are stimulated by fine needles which unblock the flow of Qi at these points. Your practitioner may use his or her fingers to manipulate the needles; or he or she may opt to use a small amount of electricity passed through the needles to stimulate a particular point.

The flow of life energy can be disturbed by many things, including illness and emotional states. Using needles as fine as a human hair, your acupuncturist will try to activate your body's energy channels, treat any disease, boost your immune system, promote your body's natural healing powers, and alleviate fatigue. Because it is safe and effective, with no known side effects, even those who feel a little nervous about needles may find acupuncture an effective option.

Acupuncture has been shown to ease disturbances of the digestive, hormonal, and circulatory systems. It has provided some people relief from structural and inflammatory problems such as arthritis, trauma, and back pain—all causes of recurring head pain.

In addition to treating specific problems, another bonus of acupuncture is that it may strengthen the body generally. It can help to stimulate the immune system and has a beneficial effect on the circulation, blood pressure, heart rhythm, and the secretion of gastric juices. It may also stimulate a variety of hormones that help the body respond more efficiently to injury and stress.

By treating underlying imbalances in the body, acupuncture over the long term can cure people. But it also has a short-term effect. Many patients find swift relief from symptoms after a session of acupuncture, since the needles, when properly placed, seem to activate the body's own painkilling chemicals. This is one reason why acupuncture has been used successfully in patients undergoing surgery and also to reduce the pain of giving birth.

The way acupuncture works to relieve headaches is not entirely clear. It does not appear to increase levels of endorphins—the body's natural painkillers. Levels of these endorphins may be low in migraine sufferers anyway, and studies which tried to find out whether acupuncture can raise endorphin levels have not been successful. Acupuncture appears to increase the levels of another chemical, serotonin—which enhances our feelings of well-being and also regulates the diameter of blood vessels.

In general, studies using acupuncture for headaches have been encouraging. Over an eight-month period in New Zealand, a small group of people who had experienced severe, regular migraines for more than five years showed positive results after being treated by acupuncture. In that study, acupuncture was compared to a placebo as well as to an analgesic, naloxone. Acupuncture was found to have the most significant effect, with forty percent of the subjects showing a fifty to one hundred percent reduction in the number and duration of their headaches. Although the subjects' sensation of pain was not altered, attacks were less severe and the common nausea and vomiting were not always present in their migraine attacks.

Another study concluded that electroacupuncture was most effective in treating muscle contraction headaches. Of 177 patients with long-term, chronic head and face pain, acupuncture reduced pain in fifty-six percent of the group. Two years later, researchers found that forty-seven percent of those who had improved had elected to carry on with the treatment on a long-term basis, and were experiencing periods of relief of up to two years. Moreover, twenty-one percent had discontinued treatment because they no longer got attacks of migraine.

In a study comparing acupuncture to the beta-blocker drug metoprolol, acupuncture was shown to be at least as effective in reducing the frequency and duration of attacks (though not their severity), and superior in terms of negative side effects. Other studies comparing acupuncture with conventional treatment have found similar results.

ACUPRESSURE

If you are still not convinced, or simply don't like the idea of needles, acupressure, which works on the same points but using finger pressure instead of needles, can also be helpful for most headaches. Unlike acupuncture, acupressure does not need to be applied by a professional—the simple techniques can be learned by anyone. Those who follow this discipline believe that pain almost anywhere in the body can be relieved within minutes by using the Asian self-help technique called G-jo acupressure. G-jo means first aid in Chinese. There are at least twenty important acupoints for relieving the many types of headaches that Western medicine has identified. Fortunately, you do not need to learn them all, since there are several broadly acting points on the body which can produce immediate, often miraculous, results. Two points are particularly useful for headaches:

1. G-jo 13, which is in the webbing between the thumb and forefinger. To find it, squeeze the two together, place a finger atop the fleshy mound that is formed. Keep your finger on the mound and relax your hand. Then begin to stimulate the point, first with deep pressure and after a few seconds with a kind of digging massage. The more this place hurts, the more it is likely to be the right place for you to stimulate during a headache. Avoid stimulating this point during pregnancy.
2. G-jo 4 is located on the arm in line with the middle finger. To find it, bend your wrist backward and measure two thumb widths above the most prominent crease in your upper wrist. You should feel a slight hollow in between the two bones of the arm. Relax your wrist, find the tender spot, and stimulate it in the same way as G-jo 13 for a few seconds.

When stimulating these two points, you may have to press for a minute or so (no more). Once you have done one side, then do the other. Always release the pressure when a change occurs in your symptoms; your body will then take over the healing process.

Occasionally you may experience minor reactions when

applying these simple, self-help techniques. These can include a slight flush or perspiration across the brow or shoulders; indeed you may feel warmth and clamminess anywhere on the body. These are normal reactions and pass quickly. Most people report a profound sense of relief after stimulating the right acupoint.

CHAPTER 10

Hypnotherapy

Hypnotherapy induces a trance-like state that enables an individual to explore the deepest levels of his or her mind, body, and emotions. While in a hypnotic trance, positive suggestions can then be made and heard at a very deep level to help bring about change in the patient. Hypnotherapy is so effective it has been used by dentists and doctors in lieu of anesthetics. There is even a case of a fifteen-year-old girl undergoing a heart operation without anesthesia while under hypnosis.

Hypnosis is one of the oldest forms of therapy. Ancient writings confirm that the Sumerian healers gave sufferers hypnotic suggestions. Hindu fakirs, Persian magi, and Indian yogi also used hypnotic suggestions. The Ebers papyrus tells us that ancient Egyptian priest-doctors would ask sufferers to fix their gaze upon a glossy piece of metal to help induce a trance-like state. It's a technique which is still commonly used by modern practitioners.

Today, ninety-four percent of patients say they have derived some benefit from hypnotherapy. Relaxation is the most commonly reported effect. It has been used to treat a wide range of conditions including headache, respiratory problems, sleep disorders, stress, and chronic pain.

The mind is divided into two parts, the conscious and unconscious. Some practitioners liken it to an iceberg: the conscious mind is the tip, the unconscious is the large mass lying beneath the surface. What lurks in the unconscious is often at the root of our health problems, since the body and mind are constantly interacting in ways which the conscious mind is not aware of.

In order to function on a day-to-day basis, we need to remain on a conscious level. But this does not mean that we should avoid the unconscious. A number of people find the idea of confronting the unconscious frightening—almost like having to walk down a dark, unfamiliar street in the dead of night. However, the unconscious isn't just a chaotic jumble of scary memories and dark secrets. It also holds our potential for good, as well as our under-used creativity and richest emotions. For many people, hypnotherapy is a way to access the good as well as the unfamiliar and scary. Hypnotherapy is a way to address these things in a safe, controlled way.

Hypnosis is not the same as sleep. When the brain waves of hypnotized subjects have been monitored, alpha wave activity is increased. These are the electrical impulses which are produced when humans are relaxed but mentally alert. When a person is asleep, this is not the case: slower delta waves are the predominant type of brain activity.

For hypnosis to work, you must want to be hypnotized. Your willingness to take this step opens the door to a dialogue with your unconscious self. People who have lived with headaches for years often forget what it is like to live without pain. The pain has become so deeply ingrained, it is viewed as part of their personality. They may even believe, on some level, that they need pain in order to make them feel alive. One benefit of hypnosis is that it can take you back to a time when you were pain free so that you re-experience what that was like. It can provide positive, supportive suggestions which can help you create new, pain-free patterns in your life. For instance, if your headache is a response to stress, you can begin to build new, more positive responses to help you deal with stress.

There is a good deal of evidence to suggest that hypnosis, although it works primarily on the mind, produces a number of profound physical effects, including slower heartbeat and breathing rate, dilation of the bronchi in the lungs, lowered blood pressure, and more efficient production of stomach acid. It is also thought that hypnotherapy can strengthen the immune system, making it an ideal tool for treating a range of health disorders, such as tension headaches and other stress-related problems.

You can contact a hypnotherapist, or you can do the work yourself. It is particularly useful for headaches which stem from stress, anxiety, or depression. For instance, when researchers from Brigham and Women's Hospital in Boston, Massachusetts used hypnotherapy to ease chronic tension headaches, they discovered that the duration and intensity of these headaches were significantly reduced. In another study, hypnotherapy was shown to be three times more effective in producing complete remission of the symptoms of migraine than the conventional drug prochlorperazine (Stemetil). In children from six to twelve years old who had classic migraines but had received no previous treatments, a comparison of self-hypnosis with the drug propranolol showed that while self-hypnosis did not alter the severity of the attacks, it did reduce the number.

In one study, researchers were puzzled as to why some patients improved and others did not. They concluded that merely your act of seeking out an alternative therapy often represents a commitment to yourself and your own well-being. Those people who acknowledged their need for help and persisted in seeking appropriate treatment (in this case, learning and applying self-hypnosis) experienced longer-term relief. Later, some of the researchers from this same group went on to study whether it was possible to predict which patients would experience pain reduction through hypnosis. They started to study outside factors such as their health status and psychological profile. They found that those who were confident of a cure before treatment achieved greater pain reduction—a phenomenon not unknown in other areas of medicine.

If you are seeing a hypnotherapist, the chances are that he or she will give you some self-hypnosis suggestions which you can practice at home. These usually encourage you to take a few moments each day to relax and reinforce the positive suggestions that you received during your formal session.

Anyone can practice simple self-hypnosis at any time. You need to be somewhere quiet where you can be assured of few distractions. You should be sitting comfortably in a chair. You should also be clear about what you would like to achieve, for example, complete relaxation of your tense muscles, letting go of obsessive thoughts, or steadying your nerves. Begin by focusing on a point in front of you. It can be anything—a picture, a pattern on the wallpaper, a place where the light is reflected on the wall. Let everything except that object drop away from your mind. Stare at the object until you begin to see it change. That's the signal to close your eyes. Now let your attention come to your body. Pick somewhere in your body that you are particularly aware of at that moment. It could be your eyelids or the way your lungs are taking in air, it could even be your aching head. Let everything else drop away and focus on that point in your body until you feel a change: your breathing may slow down, or a tense muscle may begin to relax.

Once you reach this stage, you can help yourself go into a deeper trance by counting backward from ten to zero. Some people like to imagine that they are descending a staircase and that with each step they are becoming more relaxed and receptive. Using the opposite method, counting up and ascending the staircase, is a gentle way of coming out of hypnosis.

When you are in this trance-like state, try to find as many ways as you can to say the same positive things to yourself. It may help to write them out beforehand. Instead of "I will not be tense," try "I am relaxed and calm." Instead of "I won't let the pressure get on top of me," say "I am coping well with all the things I have to do."

Try also to make good use of your imagination. If you are tense about something you have to do at work, imagine yourself coping with confidence at each stage of the day: getting up, traveling to work, arriving at work, seeing your colleagues, attending meetings, and so on. Explore all the possibilities of the day and your reactions to them, reminding yourself at each stage that you are coping in a relaxed and positive way.

Remember that negative patterns take a long time to build up and an equally long time to knock down. Doing this type of exercise once or twice is unlikely to produce great results. You will need to practice each day for a month or more to begin to feel a change in yourself and in the way you respond to outside forces. Like many alternative therapies, hypnotherapy requires a commitment to yourself and your own well-being. It also requires a commitment of time in order to restructure the less positive aspects of your personality and to bring out your best qualities.

CHAPTER 11

Osteopathy and Chiropractic Care

When headaches are the result of neck injury or strain, osteopathy or chiropractic intervention is often of great benefit. Osteopathy and chiropractic care evolved around the same time largely along the same lines. Both osteopaths and chiropractors believe that subtle and not-so-subtle misalignments of the body can result in illness. Because of this, people who consult either type of practitioner often come to rely on them to treat a range of health problems.

OSTEOPATHY

Osteopathy can be used on its own or in conjunction with conventional treatments. It is a hands-on therapy. The practitioner is concerned with the relationship between the muscles and skeletal system and the way in which the body functions.

However, many osteopaths see their roles as more than just fixing mechanical dysfunction. Many osteopaths are interested not only in the structure of the spine;, but the subtle movement of energy through the body as well, and how this movement of energy affects the mind, body, and emotions. Therefore, some practitioners will undertake the treatment of respiratory, gastrointestinal, and cardiovascular problems by aiming to restore the free flow of vital energy to these areas.

Other osteopaths believe osteopathy to be effective for stress, anxiety, and depression. In addition, some osteopaths are trained in both osteopathy and naturopathy and will approach their practice from a more holistic, naturopathic point of view. Clearly, the way one osteopath works may be very different than another. Therefore, it is important to discuss what conditions your practitioner prefers to treat before you begin.

Osteopaths work with their hands, some applying pressure gently on the soft tissues or scalp. This technique is called cranial osteopathy and is particularly suitable to young children. Some will use rhythmic movement and occasionally more forceful techniques to mobilize stiff joints.

CHIROPRACTIC CARE

Chiropractic care developed around the same time as osteopathy and is used to treat the same kinds of musculoskeletal problems. Nevertheless, there are subtle differences in the approach chiropractors take. Chiropractic care concerns itself mostly with the spinal column and the effects of misalignments of the spinal joints. Chiropractors believe that misalignment of these joints can result in poor health in the nervous system and the organs of the body.

In chiropractic care, the spinal column is of supreme importance, since it acts as a kind of switchboard for the rest of the body. If bones move out of place due to soft tissue damage, allergies, sensitivities, tension, or toxic build-up, the nerves are affected and chronic illness and pain such as headaches, digestive disturbances, PMS, and emotional problems can result.

Chiropractic care is more commonly practiced in the

United States, where there are over 55,000 practitioners treating an estimated 15 to 20 million patients each year. In the United Kingdom, osteopathy is the more popular therapy.

Tension headaches can particularly benefit from treatment by an osteopath or chiropractor. In America, the National Institutes of Health have concluded that chiropractic manipulation is better than drugs for the long-term management of chronic headaches. Chiropractic research, for instance, estimates that once the cause of the headache is identified, around eighty percent of those treated can experience long-term benefits after just a few short sessions.

Both osteopaths and chiropractors will take a full history from you and discuss the nature of your headache. They may ask you questions about whether you sit for prolonged periods at work or at home, check your posture, and ask about previous injuries which may have involved the head, neck, spine, or joints.

If your headache has a structural or postural root, the chiropractor or osteopath can help realign your body and release tension. If your structural problem is caused by something other than soft tissue damage, your practitioner may recommend that you follow a complementary regime to maintain your health. This may involve altering your diet or using herbs to flush toxins out of your system and improve immune system function.

There is some reluctance by conventional medicine to admit that manipulation can help relieve headaches. For instance, one major American study of chiropractic research from 1966 to the present day tried to assess how effective it was in the treatment of neck pain and headache. The researchers scanned four computerized databases and retrieved 134 studies for analysis. After a review of the evidence, which showed that spinal manipulation provided short-term benefits for some, had only a low rate of complications, and compared favorably with the use of muscle relaxants, the authors only grudgingly concluded that chiropractic might be of use in some cases.

The benefits of spinal manipulation over conventional drugs can be observed in other studies. In another U.S. study, 150 subjects with chronic tension headaches were randomly assigned to receive either 10–30 mg of the antidepressant/sedative amitriptyline at bedtime for six weeks, or chiropractic treatment twice weekly for six weeks. Results showed that while both groups improved at similar rates at first, a follow-up consultation four weeks after the treatment ceased showed that only the chiropractic group were experiencing continued relief from their headache pain. In this study, more than eighty percent of the drug group reported side effects such as drowsiness, dry mouth, and weight gain, as opposed to around four percent in the manipulation group who reported neck soreness and stiffness as the main side effects. Again, the conclusion was somewhat grudging. The authors suggested that because of small numbers, the study was not conclusive and that further studies should account for the placebo effect (in other words, the ability of a placebo to provide a cure for some people) of the doctor-patient relationship. One wonders when medical research will also control for the nocebo effect (the ability of a doctor's attitude, personality, and beliefs to negatively influence his patient's health) of the doctor-patient relationship!

Perhaps one of the biggest benefits of spinal manipulation is that it can help reduce your intake of painkillers. Since the overuse of these has been associated with a number of health problems, including stomach upsets and rebound headaches, this is a real plus. In one small study of patients suffering from chronic headache, half received spinal manipulation twice weekly and the other half received laser treatment combined with deep friction massage twice a week for three weeks. Researchers found that while the use of painkillers decreased by thirty-six percent in the spinal manipulation group, it remained unchanged in the massage group. The number of headaches per day also decreased, by sixty-nine percent in the manipulation group compared with only thirty-six percent in the massage group. Headache intensity also decreased by thirty-six percent in the spinal manipulation group compared with a seventeen percent decrease in the massage group.

If you are seeking osteopathic or chiropractic help, you will probably get the best results if you combine this with self-help. For instance, it is no good having your spine realigned if you are just going to go back to sitting in the same unsupported, uncomfortable chair or sleeping on the same sagging mattress day after day, or if you continue to adopt a posture which throws your spine and joints right back out again.

If your diet is inadequate or poor, it may be contributing to chronic musculoskeletal problems. Regimes such as the Alexander Technique are particularly good in helping postural problems, and regular yoga will help keep your joints flexible. Without this kind of commitment, osteopathy and chiropractic care may be able to provide only Band-Aid therapy. As with any alternative therapy, patients have to make changes in their personal lifestyle in order to support the return to good health.

— CHAPTER **12** —

Aromatherapy

Throughout history, volatile oils extracted from flowers, herbs, and animal sources have been used to calm or stimulate the emotions, and enhance well-being. Our sense of smell is the sense most directly linked to the emotional centers of the brain; pleasing smells can lift moods and have been known to alleviate certain symptoms, such as headache pain.

There are about 150 essential oils which are distilled from plants, flowers, trees, bark, grasses, and seeds, each with its distinctive therapeutic, psychological, and physiological effect. Some are antiseptic, others are anti-viral, anti-inflammatory, pain-relieving, antidepressant, and expectorant. They can be used to stimulate, relax, improve digestion, and eliminate excess water.

Essential oils should always be derived from natural sources. The cosmetic industry long ago abandoned the use of genuinely natural ingredients and bases its products today on fragrances derived from petrochemicals. These fragrances are used in cosmetics and household products as well as in foods, where they are called flavors or aromas. Flavors and aromas are also used heavily in the tobacco industry to enhance the flavor of cigarettes, especially in the lower tar and nicotine brands.

Synthetic oils do not work the same way as natural oils and may produce a range of undesired effects. Numerous bath preparations in particular say they contain natural ingredients such as citrus or lavender. What they really mean is that they contain chemical fragrances which approximate the smell of these natural substances.

Studies have shown that inhaling synthetic fragrances can cause negative circulatory changes in the brain. Subtle negative changes in electrical activity in the brain can also occur with exposure to petrochemical fragrances. These types of fragrances are a frequent trigger of migraine headaches. When you are buying an essential oil, always make sure that the manufacturer has put the Latin name on the label; otherwise, you could be buying a synthetic oil or a mixture of oils derived from natural and synthetic oils made from petrochemicals.

Aromatherapy is suitable for self-help and is widely used in homes, clinics, and hospitals in a variety of applications. They can be used in baths or steam inhalations, sprinkled on pillows or sheets, used in oil burners, diffusers, and vaporizers. When aromatherapy is combined with massage it can have a profound effect on an individual's sense of well-being. Massage with essential oils is not only pleasant, it can help boost immunity—thus reducing the risk of contracting viral infections associated with headaches.

Massage also has a psychological effect. Therapeutic touch has long been good medicine for those suffering from anxiety and depression.

Different oils work in different ways. Most work indirectly to relieve pain; lavender oil, for instance, can be used for relaxation and sound sleep. One oil in particular, peppermint, has been shown to work directly to relieve pain. It is thought that peppermint oil possesses analgesic properties and works in part by stimulating the nerve fibers which register cold. This in turn reduces the pain information transmitted to the brain.

In trials with headache sufferers, peppermint was combined with similar oils such as eucalyptus to gauge which combination was most effective for headaches. The most effective combinations found were those where peppermint was the dominant oil. For instance, while equal amounts of peppermint and eucalyptus increased subjects' mental agility and had a muscle- and mind-relaxing effect, peppermint with traces of eucalyptus was shown to have a more significant analgesic effect, and reduced the pain of a tension headache. While peppermint is a good first choice for the direct treatment of headache pain, some headaches respond more to complex blends of oils.

The beauty of aromatherapy is that you can take part in the process of healing by selecting and blending your own oils. With a few exceptions, such as tea tree and lavender, most essential oils are simply too strong to be used neat. Therefore, always mix your oils in a base or carrier oil before you apply them to your skin or put them into your bath. Any vegetable-based oil will do as a carrier, but many people prefer lighter oils such as almond, apricot kernel, or grapeseed oil.

You can use the following table to guide you in making up your own individual blends:

Amount of Essential Oil	Amount of Base Oil
1 drop	1 ml
2–5 drops	5 ml (approx. 1 tsp.)
4–10 drops	10 ml (approx. 1 dessertspoon)

Amount of Essential Oil cont.	Amount of Base Oil cont.
6–15 drops	15 ml (approx. 1/2 oz. or 1 tbs.)
8–20 drops	20 ml
10–25 drops	25 ml
12–30 drops	30 ml (approx. 1 oz.)

Now, consider some of the following suggestions for pleasant relief from different sources of headache pain.

INSOMNIA

Since anxiety, stress, and lack of sleep are often linked to chronic headaches, anything which reduces these triggers should also act to reduce the frequency of headaches. It is certainly worth considering using aromatherapy to help you sleep. Instead of taking sleeping pills, try altering the atmosphere of your room with the scent of lavender.

In one study of patients suffering from long-term insomnia, sedatives were withdrawn and lavender oil was used as an "ambient odor." (In other words, a diffuser was used to scent the air with lavender.) Not only did the patients report getting more sleep, they reported better sleep. Lavender oil was shown to be as effective as medication, without any of the unpleasant side effects. What is more, lavender oil helped reduce the restless, troubled sleep which sometimes comes as a result of insomnia.

During the day, try mixing lavender with uplifting oils such as geranium, clary sage, lemon, neroli, and Roman chamomile.

STRESS AND ANXIETY

In her book *The Fragrant Mind*, internationally renowned aromatherapist Valerie Ann Worwood suggests that all stresses are not equal. In order to find relief from anxiety and stress, you will need to dig a little deeper and identify your individual responses to stress. Once identified, you can try any of these combinations to help ease the tension. These essential oil combinations should be mixed in approximately 30 ml (1 ounce) of base oil.

- For tense anxiety with symptoms of bodily tension and muscle aches and pain try mixing 10 drops of clary sage, 15 drops of lavender, and 5 drops of Roman chamomile.
- For restless anxiety with symptoms such as dizziness, sweating, overactivity, heart palpitations, a lump in the throat, and stomach upsets, try 5 drops of vetiver, 10 drops of juniper, and 15 drops of cedarwood.
- For apprehensive anxiety with symptoms including worrying, brooding, unease, and a sense of foreboding, even paranoia, use 15 drops of bergamot, 5 drops of lavender, and 10 drops of geranium.
- For repressed anxiety with symptoms of edginess, lack of concentration, irritability, insomnia, or chronic exhaustion, use 10 drops each of neroli, rose otto, and bergamot.

Any of these mixtures can be used in massage, put into the bath, inhaled with steam, or put onto a warm or cool compress and applied to the head.

DEPRESSION

Many of the oils used for anxiety and stress are also effective for depression. However, for quick relief from a minor depressive state, citrus oils have been shown to be most effective. Try using mandarin, grapefruit, lemon, or orange according to your inclination. These can be used in an oil burner to alter the atmosphere of your room or in a relaxing massage. If either of these methods is not practical, if for instance, if you are traveling or at work, sprinkle some citrus essential oil on a cotton handkerchief and carry it with you in a small plastic bag. When you feel your spirits flag, you can discreetly take the hankie out and inhale deeply two or three times for a refreshing boost.

SINUSITIS

A combination of eucalyptus and menthol used as an ointment has been shown to be effective in treating the symptoms of most upper respiratory tract infections. Both oils encourage the secretion of mucus and act as anti-microbials. If you cannot find a ready-made ointment, you can mix these in a carrier oil and apply around the nose or make a steam inhalation. Other helpful oils for sinusitis include lavender, tea tree, eucalyptus, rosemary, juniper, bergamot, hyssop, cajuput, neroli, thyme, and lemon oils, singly or in combination.

TRY TIGER BALM

Although not strictly an essential oil, Tiger Balm contains a combination of essential oils which can provide quick first aid for headaches. You can purchase Tiger Balm (either the red or white formula; there is little difference, though enthusiasts swear that the red, with its addition of cinnamon oil, is stronger) in most pharmacies and health food shops. This is a surprisingly effective type of aromatherapy, which can be applied directly to the temples to ease tension headaches.

Tiger Balm contains several essential oils such as camphor, menthol, cajuput, and clove oil, which have been shown to be effective in relieving muscular strain. They also act as vasodilators, ensuring an even flow of blood through the veins. In one small but interesting Australian study, sufferers of tension headaches were given either Tiger Balm, a neutral ointment which had an added fragrance to give it a strong smell, or the headache medication acetaminophen. Sufferers were asked to record any changes in their headache pain over the course of three hours after administration of their treatment. Those using Tiger Balm reported a much greater improvement in their headaches within five minutes to two hours of using the treatment than those using the neutral ointment.

What is really interesting, however, is that after three hours there was no difference in the level of reduction of pain between the Tiger Balm users and those who took acetaminophen. In fact, Tiger Balm delivered quicker relief, within five to fifteen minutes of using it. So Tiger Balm was better in the short term and equal to conventional drugs after three hours—and has no side effects. Given this, which would you rather take?

CHAPTER 13

Children's Headaches

While children's headaches have the same causes as those experienced by adults, their treatment may require a little more sensitivity. A child with a limited vocabulary may be unable to describe how his or her head feels. Ask most young children where it hurts and they are likely to point to their tummies—and indeed, migraines in young children may be felt in the abdomen. While the vast majority of children's headaches can be safely treated at home or with the help of alternative therapies, parents may need to listen very carefully in order to diagnose the cause and thus find the appropriate treatment for their child.

Like adults, children's headaches generally follow a pattern, though there are some differences in the type of headache and their patterns as experienced by children. One reason for these differences is that children suffer from a range of illnesses that are different from adults. Children are unlikely to have neck injuries, although osteopaths would argue that obstetrically managed birth, which is not generally gentle, often constitutes a trauma to the neck and head. They will not suffer from menstrual difficulties, strokes, or high blood pressure. Children do have more fevers and a wider range of completely new viral and bacterial infections that their immature immune systems must learn to deal with; they may have more eye and tooth problems as well.

For children, the world, full of teachers, bullies, marital disharmony, sibling rivalry, TV, and videos, presents a very frightening view of life and is more emotionally challenging than the world adults faced as children. Not surprisingly, many children experience their first headaches around the age of four—just about the time they first enter school. Going to school is potentially emotionally upsetting and exhausting—many children are in school hours longer than most adults work during the day. It is also the time when children, under pressure from their peers, begin eating more junk food such as chocolate, chips, and sugary drinks. This is also when sports and extracurricular activities become more common. But even activities that are fun can be overdone and cause fatigue—not surprisingly, the most common type of headache children get is the tension headache.

Young children can also suffer from migraines, but again the pattern is somewhat different than it is for adults. While adult migraine is more common in women, in children under twelve migraine is more common in boys. It is only from puberty on that girls suffer from headaches more than boys. Children who have headaches lose more than twice the number of school days than children who do not.

Often children complaining of headaches are not given the consideration they deserve. In one Finnish study of nearly 1,000 children around the age of seven, around twenty percent of children experienced headaches severe enough to disrupt their daily activities at least once in their lives. Less than a quarter of these children had been taken to a doctor to investigate the headache, and only a small percentage of those children with migraine had been diagnosed before the study.

This study yielded some interesting information about the causes of children's headaches. For example, most started in the afternoon and were made worse by physical activity. The researchers also found that children who have headaches were more likely to grind their teeth at night and thus report tenderness around the jaw and in the neck muscles.

POTENTIALLY DANGEROUS HEADACHES

Though rare, headaches can sometimes be symptoms of a serious problem such as meningitis. You should call a doctor if your child's headache:

- Is accompanied by fever, vomiting, stiff neck, lethargy, or confusion
- Follows a head injury
- Occurs in the morning accompanied by nausea
- Increases in severity over the course of a day or from one day to the next
- Is suddenly brought on by a sneeze or a cough
- Interferes with school or other activities
- Is restricted to one side of the head

Whatever the cause, children's headaches should always be taken seriously. Not because they are a sign that something is seriously wrong—this is rarely the case—but because children are much less adept at handling pain than adults. They don't rationalize it away; all they know is that it hurts and they want somebody or something to make it better.

It is particularly important with children to avoid providing a pill for every pain. This introduces a very poor attitude to health and illness at a young and vulnerable age. Instead, try some of the following suggestions:

- Quiet things down. Try not to load your child's schedule up with lots of activities—however convenient it may be for you. Instead, every day should have a time when your child can paint or play quietly. Better still, use this time to play quietly or read with your child.
- Talk to your child. If the headache seems to be in response to emotional tension, try to discover the source and deal with it. Just letting your child know you care is good medicine, since sometimes tension headaches are cries for attention.
- Give your child some control over his or her day-to-day life. Children, like adults, are more prone to headaches when they feel out of control and pushed around. If your child is stressed out or has a problem, don't try to fix it for him or her. Instead, encourage a dialogue where your child can come up with his or her own unique solutions.
- Rub it away. If the muscles around the temples are tender, gently rubbing them can bring relief. If they are too tender and your child says stop, then stop. But many children simply like being touched and stroked gently by their parents. If your child gets a stomachache headache, try rubbing the abdomen gently in a clockwise direction. Children also respond well to foot massage.
- Keep their blood sugar up with sensible foods. Make sure breakfasts are nourishing and that lunches actually get eaten instead of traded away or thrown in the trash. Skipping a meal can bring on a headache or make an existing one worse in some children.

- Cut out caffeine. Your child's headache could be a rebound headache caused by the caffeine in sodas and chocolates. These are empty foods anyway and should be restricted to an occasional treat.
- Use the G-jo acupressure technique recommended on page 97.
- If the headache persists, have your child lie down in a darkened room with a cool aromatherapy compress on the forehead.
- Consider homeopathy. This is probably a safer alternative than herbs, especially for very young children. Children rarely need the most potent remedies, so for self-treatment stick to 6c potencies and give one tablet every half-hour for up to four hours during headache attacks until the pain begins to ease. Try Valeriana officianalis or Passiflora to induce sleep and relieve anxiety; Chamomilla to calm frayed nerves; Kali bromatum for fearfulness and nervousness; Carbo veg or Silica for digestive disturbances; Pulsatilla for weepiness and changeability; or Calc phos for headaches caused by emerging teeth.

Children are as prone to stress as adults. Studies into relaxation techniques have had variable results, but the overall trend is positive. In one American study, children who were diagnosed as suffering from tension headaches used a combination of relaxation and biofeedback. In this study more than half of the children experienced at least a 50 percent improvement in the frequency and severity of their headaches. Other studies have shown similarly good results.

Visualization and meditation can be useful in children who are still comfortable using their imagination. Simple relaxation skills can be taught by parents at home. Sit quietly with your children and ask them to imagine they are in a warm shower and that anyplace the water strikes their bodies instantly feels more relaxed. Stay with this image for as long as it takes for your child to relax. A similarly helpful guided image is to suggest that your children picture stepping into a warm pool where the water gradually rises over their toes, feet, ankles, and gradually upward. Ask your children to imagine that as the water touches their bodies, the muscles gently relax and the pain floats away. This is a form of progressive muscle relaxation which children will find less boring than formal progressive relaxation (and it's a good guided imagery for adults too).

Inevitably, some parents and children will feel awkward taking time to relax. It is amazing how little patience we have for doing nothing. Don't nag your children if they don't do the exercises on their own. Talking to them about headache pain and the benefits of learning to relax is a better approach. Better yet, if you want to get your children to use relaxation techniques, practice with them. It will probably do you both good.

You can further help by structuring space and time in the day for your child to relax. Instead of forcing your children to relax (which of course defeats the purpose!), let them know that they should want to be doing it for themselves—and make it clear that you want to help them succeed. Most children will go along with this because it gives them control over the situation.

In one of the most thorough trials to date on children's headaches, food allergy, and the frequency of migraine, conducted by the Department of Neurology at London's Great Ormond Street Hospital and published in the medical journal *The Lancet* in 1983, researchers discovered that ninety-three percent of the children in the trial—children who suffered from severe, frequent migraine—recovered once the foods they were allergic to had been detected and eliminated from their diet. The most common allergens were the same as those listed in Chapter 5.

A recent study in a professional journal dedicated to the study of pain showed that children's headaches can be caused by a variety of obvious factors. Chief among these were fatigue and lack of sleep. Fatigue and sleep deprivation were also leading causes of both tension and migraine headaches in the Finnish research discussed earlier.

To help your children sleep well, you can use gentle remedies such as sprinkling lavender oil on their pillows. Another good way to help them unwind before bedtime is to give them a warm bath with soothing essential oils in it. Make sure that the hour or so before bed is always quiet and be as firm and regular about bedtimes as you can. Although most children will balk at one time or another about bedtime, the more it becomes a matter of routine, the less trouble they will have dropping off.

CHAPTER 14

Everyday Remedies

Over the years, many different folk remedies have evolved to give quick relief to headache pain. Some are more effective than others, and while these will not address the root cause of your headache, they may help to ease the pain and get you back on track quickly. You may have to experiment to find the remedy which suits you best.

Many of the ingredients are those which you have at hand at home.

BRUSH YOUR HAIR

Brushing your hair each day isn't just a vanity. It can help to improve the circulation in your scalp and reduce the occurrence of headache. Use a natural bristle brush or one with rounded tips and brush your hair in a downward motion. You can also give yourself a mini-massage by brushing in small circles, beginning at your temples and working your way down from your scalp. Make sure you cover all of your scalp in this way for the greatest benefit.

MAKE A COMPRESS

Cool and warm compresses on the head can be very restful and revitalizing. All you need is a washcloth and a few ingredients commonly found in the kitchen. Soak your washcloth in one of the three following mixtures. Combined with a twenty-minute rest, this should help lift your headache.

Ginger Compress

Cut and peel one whole root of fresh ginger. Boil it in 3 cups of water until it turns cloudy. Soak your washcloth in the warm mixture and then apply it to the back of your neck. This works to expand the contracted muscles and relieve dull, steady pain.

Vinegar Compress

Soak your washcloth in vinegar and place it in the refrigerator until it is sufficiently chilled. Apply to your forehead, neck, and temples. You can also inhale vinegar for quick relief. To do this, boil equal parts of vinegar and water, and pour the mixture into a bowl or basin; place a towel over the bowl and your head and inhale the beneficial steam.

Herbal Compress

Almost any aromatic herb tea can be good for this, but ideally you should boil 3 cups of water and pour it over 1 tablespoon of lavender and 1 tablespoon of chamomile. Steep for 20 minutes. Soak your washcloth in the mixture, wring it out, and apply on the back of the neck and/or forehead. This mixture is equally effective warm or cool.

TREAT YOUR FEET

Draw congestion away from your head with a warming foot bath. Put 1 tablespoon of powdered mustard or ginger in a basin big enough for both of your feet. Fill the basin with water as hot as you can bear; sit in a comfortable chair and slowly immerse your feet in the water. You can drape a towel over the basin to keep the heat in. Placing a cool washcloth on your forehead or neck will also help.

Alternatively, try an icy foot bath. Fill a basin with icy water and soak your feet in it. After a few minutes, your feet will start to feel warm and your headache may drain away.

HOT AND COLD

Alternating hot and cold showers will help improve your circulation and avert the vascular type headaches caused by the dilation and then constriction of the blood vessels. You should aim to do this each day, or better yet, twice a day for two or three months to help improve your circulation.

If you are away from home and can't jump into a shower, try alternating hot and cold water on your wrists. If you do this as soon as you feel a headache coming on, it may avert a full-blown headache.

MAKE A TONIC

There are two effective tonics commonly used for headache sufferers. The first is made from small pieces of ginger root, coriander seeds, and diced garlic. Put these in a pan, bring to a boil, and keep boiling until half the liquid is gone. What is left is a concentrated mixture which you can sip periodically throughout the day. Sweeten with honey if you prefer.

For headaches caused by digestive imbalances, an apple cider vinegar tonic can be helpful. Apple cider vinegar (be sure not to use any other kind) is pH neutral and has a long history of use in folk medicine. You can make a simple tonic of a glass of water with 2 teaspoons of apple cider vinegar added to it.

Have this each day with 2 teaspoons of honey to follow if you prefer.

GO NUTS

Try eating a handful of unpeeled almonds. They contain the natural "aspirin" salicin, a remedy which is used in areas of North Africa and Asia where almond trees are common.

RELIEF IN A BAG

Some people find relief from breathing into a paper bag for fifteen or twenty minutes. The carbon dioxide you inhale when breathing your "old" air can help avert vascular headaches. Try to lie down for twenty minutes afterward, especially if you feel dizzy.

APPENDIX

HEADACHES AT A GLANCE

Type of Headache	What Kind of Pain?	Main Symptoms
Tension	Steady, dull aching. Builds up gradually. Like a band around the head.	Spreads from the back of the neck, to the whole head. Head feels heavy. Does not usually throb.
Migraine	Generally one-sided, centered above or behind one eye. Pulsating, throbbing—often in time with the pulse. Drilling. Can last 2 to 72 hours.	Moderate to intense pain. Tingling in hands and face, nausea and vomiting. Classic migraine is preceded by an aura with visual disturbances. Balance and mental function are affected.
Cluster	Stabbing, one-sided. Similar to migraine. Individual attack lasts 15 minutes to 3 hours.	Comes in cycles over a period of days. Pain is behind one eye with reddening and weepiness in that eye. Facial flushing, drooping eyelids, sweating, nasal congestion.
Rebound	Comes in steady jolts. Throbbing pain can be similar to migraine.	Usually the whole head. Can begin at the back of neck and spread to entire head or just to one side.
Eyestrain	Like a tension headache. Mild steady pain. Can be felt as a pressure on the top or around the head.	Commonly located in the forehead and face. Occasionally at the back of the head or neck.
Dental	Dull, steady pain, usually felt as pressure, on the top of the head. There may be a clicking sound in the jaw.	Usually on both sides of the head, like wearing a tight headband. Tenderness around the jaw and mouth.

Brought On/Made Worse By	Best Treatments
Straining the neck and shoulder muscles. High blood pressure, stress of any kind, poor posture, food intolerance and allergy, long car journeys, computer work.	Acupuncture, aromatherapy, chiropractic, dietary and environmental changes, homeopathy, hypnotherapy, osteopathy.
Activity, light, loud noises, stress, food intolerance or allergy.	Acupuncture, aromatherapy, chiropractic, dietary and environmental changes, herbal medicine, homeopathy, hypnotherapy, osteopathy.
Seasonal changes, food intolerance and allergy, hormonal imbalance, alcohol, restless sleep, smoking.	Acupuncture, chiropractic, diet and environmental changes, herbal medicine, homeopathy, osteopathy.
Overuse of pain medications, prescription drugs, and stimulants such as caffeine, MSG, and artificial sweeteners. Psychological stress, food intolerance or allergy, chemical sensitivity.	Acupuncture, dietary and environmental changes, herbal medicine, homeopathy, hypnosis, hypnosis.
Overuse of eyes, made worse by metabolic imbalances, emotional/psychological stress, hormonal imbalance. Occasionally digestive disturbances or musculoskeletal problems.	Acupuncture, aromatherapy, dietary and environmental changes, homeopathy, osteopathy.
Faulty bite, tooth decay, gum infections, grinding the teeth at night. Pain sensations can be made worse in those who are run-down or under pressure.	Acupuncture, chiropractic, corrective dentistry, homeopathy, hypnotherapy, osteopathy.

HEADACHES AT A GLANCE

Type of Headache	What Kind of Pain?	Main Symptoms
Exertion	Sharp, throbbing pain which comes on suddenly.	Can be generalized or localized anywhere in the head.
Sinus	Comes on gradually. Pain is dull, aching, throbbing, or gnawing.	Pressure in the forehead or behind the eyes and nose. Sinus area feels tender. Occasionally fever.
Trauma	Stabbing, sharp, or dull and aching pain.	Usually at the site of trauma. Can be hard to distinguish from a tension or migraine headache. Moodiness, dizziness, nausea, insomnia, fatigue, reduced concentration.
Sensitivity Allergy	Generalized head pain which can be dull, aching, or throbbing.	Pain can be anywhere

Brought On/Made Worse By	Best Treatments
In sensitive individuals any activity such as aerobics, sex, coughing, a bowel movement, or running can be a trigger. Metabolic imbalances and stress aggravate the problem.	Acupuncture, aromatherapy, dietary and environmental changes, herbal medicine, homeopathy.
Inflammation or infection in the sinuses. Food intolerance and chemical sensitivity, pollen, dust, and smoke. Psychological stress. Occasionally musculoskeletal problems and changes in atmospheric pressure will contribute.	Acupuncture, aromatherapy, chiropractic, dietary and environmental changes, herbal medicine, osteopathy. medicine, osteopathy.
Brought on by a blow to the head. But can be referred pain from another bodily injury, especially in the spinal and neck area.	Acupuncture, chiropractic, homeopathy, osteopathy.
Food intolerance or allergy, chemical sensitivity, stress, hormonal imbalance.	Acupuncture, dietary and environmental changes, herbal medicine, homeopathy.

INDEX

A

acupressure, 86–88, 110
acupuncture, 83–88
adrenaline, 37
alcohol, 26, 47, 49, 57, 82
Alexander Technique, 98
"Alice in Wonderland" syndrome, 5
allergies. *See also* allergy headaches
    cluster headaches and, 16–17
    food, 24, 45–46
    sinus headaches and, 18
allergy headaches, 16–17, 120–121
almonds, 115, 116
aluminum, 63
Alzheimer's disease, 63
amines, 45, 49–50
amitriptyline, 97
anger, 27. *See also* stress
antibiotics, 29
antidepressants, 29, 97
anti-inflammatories, 71–72
anxiety, 27–28, 91, 95. *See also* stress
    aromatherapy for, 102–103
    writing about, in journals, 39–40
appetite suppressants, 29
Aretaeus, 6
aromatherapy, 99–105, 110
arthritis, 29, 85
artificial sweeteners, 50–51
aspartame, 50–51
aspirin, 6, 8, 72
asthma, 36

B

beauty products, 66, 99

Belladona, 78
birth
    defects, 72
    giving, 38
blood
    pressure, high, 20–21, 29, 37, 85, 91
    sugar, 54, 109
    vessels, 14, 20–21, 51
bowel movements, 20
brain tumors, 21–22
breathing, 39, 40–41, 91, 93, 116
Bryonia, 78–79

C

cadmium, 64
caffeine, 26, 45, 47, 50–51, 58–59, 64
    children and, 110
    rebound headaches caused by, 21
capsaicin, 70
carbohydrates, 53–55
carpets, 61–62
Carroll, Lewis, 5
cayenne, 70
Ch'i (life energy), 83, 84
chairs, office, 13, 40, 98
chemical substances, 18, 28–29, 60–67
children's headaches, 6–7, 13–14, 95, 106–112
chiropractic care, 18, 19–20, 94–98
chocolate, 45, 47, 52
cluster headaches, 16–17, 118–119
coffee. *See* caffeine
cold medications, 29
compresses, 113–114
constipation, 12, 78–79
contraceptives, 29

mouth, bleeding from the, 22
mucus, 17–18
muscle tension, 27–28, 37

N

naloxone, 86
Natrum Mur, 79–80
naturopathy, 95
nervous system, 25–26, 64
neurotransmitters, 25
nitrates, 49, 63
norepinephrine, 25
nose, bleeding from the, 22
nutrition. *See* food; vitamins
nuts, 47–48, 116
Nux Vomica, 80

O

office chairs, 13, 40, 98
Omega fatty acids, 55–56
opium, 6
oral contraceptives, 29
organic headaches, 21–22
osteopathy, 18, 19–20, 94–98, 106

P

paper bag, breathing into a, 116
paracetamol, 20–21
pesticides, 53, 62
phenylethylamine, 52
phosphorous, 80
plastics, in the home, 65–66
pregnancy, 72
prochlorperazine, 91
prodrome phase, of migraines, 15
propranolol, 91
prostaglandins, 30
Pulsatilla, 80–81

Q

Qi (life energy), 83, 84

R

rebound headaches, 20–21, 51, 97–98, 118–119
recovery phase, of migraines, 15
referred pain, 10
relaxation, 38, 89, 110
religion, 42–43
resolution phase, of migraines, 15
rhythmic rocking, 40

S

salt, 27
Sanguinaria, 81
seasonal changes, 16. *See also* weather
self-hypnosis, 91–92
sensitivity/allergy headaches, 16–17, 120–121
Sepia, 81–82
serotonin, 14, 25–26, 50, 54
    acupuncture and, 85
    weather and, 30
sesame salt, 57
sexual activity, 20, 82
showers, hot and cold, alternating, 115
sinus headaches, 17–18, 120–121
sinusitis, 104
sleep, 37, 72, 89
    children's headaches and, 112
    headaches which are not relieved by, 22
    improved, through aromatherapy, 102, 103
smoking, 18, 64, 79, 100
sneezing, 20
spinal cord, 25, 94–98

OTHER BOOKS IN THE SERIES

Overcoming Addiction: A Common Sense Approach
By Michael Hardiman

Psychologist Michael Hardiman addresses addiction with sensitivity and clarity for both the layperson and the recovery professional. He covers addiction's signs and symptoms, explains the psychology behind it, and tells how to stop the cycle for good.

$10.95 • Paper • ISBN 1-58091-013-0

Overcoming Sleep Disorders: A Natural Approach
By Brenda O'Hanlon, foreword by Dr. Chris Idzikowski

In this thorough handbook, Brenda O'Hanlon gives a clear explanation of sleep, discusses how much sleep people actually need, and describes common sleep disorders. She gives practical advice on how to get a better night's sleep, what help is available, and the proven benefits of complementary medicines and therapies, including homeopathy, acupuncture, herbal remedies, and aromathcrapy.

$10.95 • Paper • ISBN 1-58091-014-9

Understanding and Overcoming Depression
By Tony Bates, with foreword by Paul Gilbert

In this book, Tony Bates shares his experiences in treating depression in its many forms and varying degrees, all of them serious for sufferers and their families. He highlights the key strategies that have helped people and outlines a program that both alleviates the shame around depression and provides necessary tools to aid recovery.

$10.95 • Paper • ISBN 1-58091-031-9

Healthy Pregnancy: A Natural Approach
By Pat Thomas

Pat Thomas treats pregnancy as a state of health, suggesting practical guidelines for good diet and gentle exercises while offering sensible advice for common complaints that may occur. She also addresses the mother's emotional well-being during and after pregnancy and looks at how the father's role can be enhanced to the benefit of both parents.

$10.95 • Paper • ISBN 1-58091-085-8

www.crossingpress.com

BROWSE through the Crossing Press Web site for information on upcoming titles, new releases, and backlist books including brief summaries, excerpts, author information, reviews, and more.

SHOP our store for all of our books and, coming soon, unusual, interesting, and hard-to-find sideline items related to Crossing's best-selling books!

READ informative articles by Crossing Press authors on all of our major topics of interest.

SIGN UP for our e-mail newsletter to receive late-breaking developments and special promotions from The Crossing Press.

WATCH for a new look coming soon to the Crossing Press Web site!